Get Fit and Enjoy It:

Learn effective exercise without a gym

enjoy *

Tracy Griffen

First published in Great Britain in 2020 by Griffen Fitness Ltd
3 Balfour Street
Edinburgh
EH6 5BY
www.getfitandenjoyit.com

CONTENTS

An Introduction

Welcome to your step-by-step guide to getting fit from home, with minimal equipment. Fitness fashions come and go, however what YOU need to do to get fit doesn't change with trends. Learning how to move your body optimally for fitness is a valuable life skill. It requires practise and repetition, and this is how you get fit.

I have been teaching fitness for over 15 years. I started out by riding my bicycle to clients around Edinburgh, getting them fit with minimal equipment. This proved popular, so I opened up a private fitness studio in Leith where I teach individuals how to get fit without a gym.

Regular exercise is something we all need to do to be in peak physical condition. It's not necessarily about having a small waistline or low BMI; it's more about how you feel and how much energy you have. Being physically fit means your body can do more, you can fit more into your day and it can also benefit your mental wellbeing. "Move and feel happy" sums it up in a nutshell.

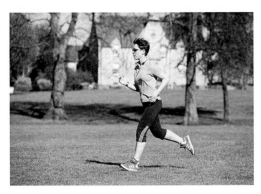

As children we naturally run about, playing and exploring the environment. As we get older, we lose that spark, that natural inquisitiveness and urge to move. Enjoying exercising is the key to making it stick. If you hate doing it, it's likely that you will do everything you can to avoid it! So part of your journey is to find forms of exercise that you enjoy and then building on it. Don't like running? You don't have to if you don't want to. But if you start with regular fast walking, you may find that in time your walking gets faster, to a jogging pace. We start at the beginning, with the simple and easy stuff.

The aim of this book is to help you incorporate more movement into your everyday life, whether it is through active commuting, fitting strength exercises into your daily routine or even just walking more – you will see the results and feel great too!

The book is structured in a similar way to how you would experience your first five Personal Training sessions at Griffen Fitness:

Before You Start: Goal setting, Medical considerations, Measurements

Week 1: Cardio exercise, Flexibility

Week 2: Strength, Abdominals (Core)

Week 3: Combining cardio / strength in a circuit

Week 4: Introducing Equipment (resistance band / exercise ball / dumbbells)

Week 5: 'Best of' workout, Measurements, Forward planning

I always chat to clients before we start in the studio to ensure we have shared expectations. There is nothing worse than a new client expecting me to act like a Drill Sergeant. Behaviour and habit change needs to be done with support and encouragement. So remember to congratulate yourself when you reach goals. It's generally recognised that it takes a month to six weeks to change a habit, and practise and repetition is important – start with the easy stuff and build up from there. It's good to start with cardio and stretching, as it's easy to learn and you can start exercising immediately.

By starting with the cardio and stretching, one can start to see results quickly. We introduce a number of strength exercises in the second week, once the cardio and stretching has been practised. Start simple, and as your fitness level improves, add intensity and more complex exercises. A bit of diary management is also required, as you'll need to remember to schedule your exercise to make sure it gets done. Write it on your list of things to do.

So, let's get started!

1. Getting Started

Fitness is like a puzzle. You need to fit all the bits together to make sure you're getting a balance. The puzzle is simple if you understand how it's put together.

The human body develops good shape when it's put under some kind of challenge. We're not designed to sit on our rears all day staring at a screen. We're made to move, and moving freely is one of the most enjoyable things about being human.

Maybe you can't move that smoothly or easily at the moment, and indeed that is what getting fit is all about. Perhaps you're thinking about the obstacles that are keeping you from getting fit: a lack of time, low mood or body confidence. Many of us have low opinions of our own bodies, this is not unusual. The best thing to do is to start moving. The method I have designed enables you to get into fitness, either for reluctant exercisers, or for those coming back from injury or illness.

The secret is to introduce a fitness programme incrementally. I'm going to guide you through how I work with PT clients in my studio. Firstly we do a medical screening questionnaire, just to check you're OK to start on an exercise programme. Here are the standard questions on a PAR-Q (Physical Activity Readiness Questionnaire):

1   Has a physician ever said you have a heart condition and you should only do physical activity recommended by a physician?

If you have a heart condition, getting fit can help. However, you need to be sure it's safe to push your heart rate up. We start with heart rate training, and wearing a heart rate monitor is a safe way to get into exercise. You will always know what your heart rate is, and can ensure that it doesn't go too high. We start aerobic exercise with walking, wearing a HRM. General medical advice is that gentle cardiovascular exercise is beneficial, but if you're unsure, or have a heart condition, please get the 'all clear' from your GP.

2   When you do physical activity, do you feel pain in your chest?

Sometimes chest pain can be related to a heart condition (see question 1), but also sometimes from muscular soreness, or tight chest muscles. It's worth having it checked out before you start.

3   Do you ever lose consciousness or do you lose your balance because of dizziness?

Dizziness can be caused by a number of things. From experience, low blood pressure seems to be the most common, but also interactions with medication and some medical conditions can contribute. If you feel dizzy at any point when exercising, stop and catch your breath. There is no need to exercise at such a high intensity that you make yourself feel awful.

4   Do you have a joint or bone problem that may be made worse by a change in your physical activity?

Lower limb issues become more common as we get older. If you've had a knee replacement, you may have been advised not to jog or to kneel. I know some people who do both after having both knees operated on, but that's their own individual decision. I prefer to err on the side of caution. Hip replacements are also not uncommon, so follow guidance. After a replacement the most important thing is to get moving as it will help the new joint 'bed in'.

5   Is a physician currently prescribing medications for your blood pressure or heart condition?

Many people with issues relating to blood pressure are prescribed medication by their GP, however it can be relatively easy to lower your blood pressure (BP) through nutrition and exercise. Doing aerobic exercise regularly will lower your BP, as does cutting out caffeine and salty foods. Less stress can help. If you're on medication your BP reading may be in the healthy zone, however you may still be unfit. Some people have side effects from BP / heart medications, so it's worth considering before embarking on an exercise programme. Always speak to your health professional before changing medications.

6   Are you pregnant?

You can still exercise, but keep it comfortable and look at it as maintaining fitness, rather than striving for new fitness goals. You can follow this programme, but you might find as the baby grows, that your heart rate increases and that everything becomes a bit more challenging. I would also advise skipping the abdominal section of the book, and try either a Pilates or pregnancy yoga class. It is advised, later in your term, to avoid prone positions (lying on your back) – many of the abdominal exercises in this book are from lying down, hence the suggestion to try a class where you can get guidance. I recommend reading the book 'Pregnancy and Fitness' by Cherry Baker, which should answer all of your questions on how to exercise safely through pregnancy.

10   Do you have insulin dependent diabetes?

If you have Type 1 Diabetes, you may find that your energy levels waver over the day. Perhaps they plummet unexpectedly. You'll probably be used to carrying some form of sugar with you. A structured exercise programme can be very helpful for you to manage your blood sugar levels. You may wish to keep an exercise diary, with comments on your blood sugar readings before and after exercise and any observations. Be sure to check with your GP if you're new to exercising and have food ready for refuelling after a workout.

8   Do you have any breathing difficulties or suffer from asthma?

Many folk with asthma are fine exercising indoors, but once they head outdoors, the Scottish chill air can trigger an asthma attack. If you have an inhaler, always have it handy (especially outdoors). If you feel wheezy, slow down or stop exercising.

9   Do you suffer from Epilepsy?

Epilepsy can involve lots of medical complications and the risk of fits during exercise. If you have epilepsy, there is no reason why you cannot exercise, however I would strongly suggest seeking the advice of your GP first and go to a highly qualified PT, discussing your requirements first.

10   Do you know of any other reason why you should not exercise or increase your physical activity?

This is really to cover all bases and ensure you're ready to go. The rule of thumb is, if you're unsure, head to your GP. You may still like to read through this book, and even take it along to your appointment to show your Doctor what your exercise plan looks like.

And Now... For Some Goal Setting

Your own personal motivation to exercise is a crucial thing to understand. Perhaps you don't actually want to exercise, but have been advised to do so by your Doctor. It might be that you can't fit into clothes you used to fit into, or maybe you've been unwell or injured and have lost your fitness over time. Or, like many, you have put on a 'Lockdown belly' from eating more and being housebound over Covid-19. Whatever the reason, have a go at answering these questions:

Are there any obstacles (i.e. job, lifestyle) in your way from increasing your fitness level?

It's good to get this out the way early. What reasons (or excuses) have you been giving yourself? Time is an issue for many people, in which case we'll be looking at quick and easy ways to fit fitness into your busy life.

Anxiety or worry about body image can be another factor. Especially if you're lacking confidence in knowing what to do. The good news is that you don't need to go to a gym to get fit. You can do it from home, and this guide will ease you into it as well. Identify potential obstacles and have a think about how they can be overcome before you even start.

Acknowledging that there are barriers (real or perceived) is part of the process of making change.

What has motivated you to become more active?

An unflattering photo, not being able to sprint for a bus, or some too-tight jeans, everyone has a different reason for wanting to get fit. The more personal and meaningful your reason, the more likely you are to succeed. Brides-to-be are often very motivated to get in shape for their special day. A SMART goal is ideal, that's a Specific, Measureable, Achievable, Relevant, Time-based goal. In other words, rather than thinking, "I'd just like to be a bit smaller", reframing the goal as "I'd like to fit into my favourite red dress for my summer holiday in July", means you're more likely to know when you've achieved it. It's easier to aim for a specific outcome, rather than a general direction.

Any specific part(s) of your body you'd like to target:

Everyone is different and some of us have a negative association with certain body parts. Sometimes someone will tell me that they "hate their bingo wings (upper arms)." One thing I find interesting is how we change our relationship with our bodies when we realise what a gift they are. When we start exercising we come to appreciate that our upper arms are actually quite important. When we learn what exercises the muscles need to do to be in good shape, we can let go of the negative view of the body part and appreciate the function.

You may wish for a part of your body to get stronger or smaller. If you have any area of your body you particularly want to focus on, it's good to recognise it early on, and also spend time figuring out exactly what it is you want from that body part. A clear visualisation of your end goal will help you stay motivated and see the results you're looking for.

What are the positive benefits you envisage from becoming more active?

It's always good to look on the bright side, as they say. Listing positive changes can help set goals as well. It's amazing how many people say that "to have more energy" is either a goal or a positive benefit. You'd think if you were doing more exercise that you would be more tired. In fact, the reverse is true. By exercising more (and eating well) you boost your metabolism. How fast you turn food into stored muscle energy has a real effect on your actual energy levels. But how do you measure someone's energy? It is quite an intangible thing. I know many people who have experienced it, miss it greatly on days they haven't been able to exercise.

In the past ten years, have you ever exercised regularly?

When was the last time you exercised? Why did you stop? If you're currently exercising, it's good to know what you're doing. That way you can adapt what you're already doing to be more effective. If you're not currently exercising, it's good to think about how long it has been since you have regularly exercised and also what has happened in the meantime. Perhaps you moved home, or jobs, developed an illness, experienced lockdown, became really busy with work... What did you do before things changed? Is that the exercise you'd like to go back to?

Do you currently exercise?

If you're currently exercising, it's good to consider what you're already doing. That way you can adapt what you're already doing to be even more effective.

Approx how many hours *daily* do you spend in front of a screen (TV / computer / phone etc)?

Add up all the hours you spend on the phone, TV, work computer, tablet etc. Then calculate your waking hours (next question), and you can see what proportion of your life is spent using a screen and therefore, probably seated. Sitting has a negative effect on the body. In short, we're not anatomically designed to sit for such a large amount of time. Our bodies were designed to stand or squat. Standing desks have become more commonplace, as we spend more and more of our time online. Simply standing up for 30 minutes a day when working can have a massive positive knock-on effect.

If you are at a computer a lot, you may like to consider your wrists. Many people have wrist pain from carpal tunnel issues without even realising it. A wrist rest or ergonomic mouse can easily alleviate the issue. Hunching over a laptop can lead to neck and shoulder pain, and tight chest muscles – have a go at some of the lying stretches in chapter 3 to ease the back.

On weekdays, what time do you usually go to bed?

This may vary between weekdays and weekends and we just want to get a general idea. You can put in a range of bedtimes if you wish. Getting to bed before midnight is important for muscle repair and general overall wellness. If you find yourself scrolling social media or staring at a screen late at night, perhaps set a phone alarm to turn off your phone at 10pm. Try and have an hour or more of 'no screen' before bed. Reading an old fashioned book is a good way to relax before bed.

What time do you wake up / get up?

You don't need to be a lark, but getting up in time for a healthy breakfast is good for mood, productivity and developing a routine. Aim to create a healthy daily routine. It may not be the same every day, but if you develop regular healthy habits you will notice an overall positive effect.

Do you prefer indoor or outdoor activities?

Worth pondering at this stage. Sometimes its weather dependent, or if you're not confident exercising in a park.

By looking at the above questions, you can put together a SMART goal. Can you imagine your goal? Visualise it in your mind's eye? Write it down....

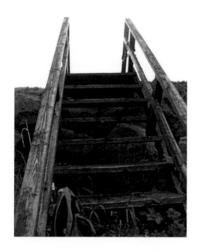

Your goal may seem out of reach, but we'll take it step-by-step

At this point in a first PT session, I would take your measurements.

We do body fat percentage. I use skinfold callipers that take a pinch from four different locations - biceps, triceps, tummy, back. I find skinfold callipers very accurate. The modern bioelectrical body fat testers that work by putting an imperceptible electric current through you can give varying readings. This is mainly because they measure your electrical resistance. Fat is more resistant than water, so the bioelectrical body fat percentage testers get different readings depending on your hydration levels.

Body Fat Classification

This is a standard classification of body fat, note that the USA has a higher % for the obese category. We all need some fat (essential fat), but too much fat can be detrimental to your health (and more weight to carry around).

Description	Women	Men
Essential Fat	10–12%	2 – 4%
Athletes	14–20%	6 – 13%
Fitness	21–24%	14 – 17%
Accceptable	25–31%	18 – 26%
Overweight / Obese (UK)	32-41%	27 – 37%
Obese (USA)	42%+	38%+

Weight

If you know your weight and height, you can calculate your BMI (Body Mass Index, see table below). This is the measurement that Doctors use, mainly as it's quick and easy to weigh a patient. In fact, body fat percentage is a better measurement of overall health. More body fat = more to carry around and therefore a greater strain on the heart and systems overall. You can be heavy through being muscular, after all, muscle is heavier and more dense than fat. It is the same for men and women. For these reasons I'm not a huge fan of BMI, but it can be interesting to see where you are on the scale:

BMI Chart

WEIGHT lbs	100	105	110	115	120	125	130	135	140	145	150	155	160	165	170	175	180	185	190	195	200	205	210	215
kgs	45.5	47.7	50.0	52.3	54.5	56.8	59.1	61.4	63.6	65.9	68.2	70.5	72.7	75.0	77.3	79.5	81.8	84.1	86.4	88.6	90.9	93.2	95.5	97.7
HEIGHT in/cm																								
5'0" - 152.4	19	20	21	22	23	24	25	26	27	28	29	30	31	32	33	34	35	36	37	38	39	40	41	42
5'1" - 154.9	18	19	20	21	22	23	24	25	26	27	28	29	30	31	32	33	34	35	36	36	37	38	39	40
5'2" - 157.4	18	19	20	21	22	22	23	24	25	26	27	28	29	30	31	32	33	33	34	35	36	37	38	39
5'3" - 160.0	17	18	19	20	21	22	23	24	24	25	26	27	28	29	30	31	32	32	33	34	35	36	37	38
5'4" - 162.5	17	18	18	19	20	21	22	23	24	24	25	26	27	28	29	30	31	31	32	33	34	35	36	37
5'5" - 165.1	16	17	18	19	20	20	21	22	23	24	25	25	26	27	28	29	30	31	32	33	34	35	35	
5'6" - 167.6	16	17	17	18	19	20	21	21	22	23	24	25	25	26	27	28	29	29	30	31	32	33	34	34
5'7" - 170.1	15	16	17	18	18	19	20	21	22	22	23	24	25	25	26	27	28	29	29	30	31	32	33	33
5'8" - 172.7	15	16	16	17	18	19	19	20	21	22	22	23	24	25	25	26	27	28	28	29	30	31	32	32
5'9" - 175.2	14	15	16	17	17	18	19	20	20	21	22	22	23	24	25	25	26	27	28	28	29	30	31	31
5'10" - 177.8	14	14	15	16	17	18	18	19	20	20	21	22	23	23	24	25	25	26	27	28	28	29	30	30
5'11" - 180.3	14	14	15	16	16	17	18	18	19	20	21	21	22	23	23	24	25	25	26	27	28	28	29	30
6'0" - 182.8	13	14	14	15	16	17	17	18	19	19	20	21	21	22	23	23	24	25	25	26	27	27	28	29
6'1" - 185.4	13	13	14	15	15	16	17	17	18	19	19	20	21	21	22	23	23	24	25	25	26	27	27	28
6'2" - 187.9	12	13	14	14	15	16	16	17	18	18	19	19	20	21	21	22	23	23	24	25	25	26	27	27
6'3" - 190.5	12	13	13	14	15	15	16	16	17	18	18	19	20	20	21	21	22	23	23	24	25	25	26	26
6'4" - 193.0	12	12	13	14	14	15	15	16	17	17	18	18	19	20	20	21	22	22	23	23	24	25	25	26

Legend: Underweight, Healthy, Overweight, Obese, Extremely obese

Women: waist and hips measurements. Using a measuring tape, measure your waist, just above your belly button. Your hips measurement is the widest part of your hips, try a few different places and make sure the tape is parallel to the ground, not hitched up on one side. Waist to hip ratio (WHR) is a useful measure of health. 'Apple shaped' women, with a larger waist to hips are more inclined to experience health issues like heart disease or type 2 diabetes. 'Pear shaped' is meant to be a healthier distribution of fat. Fat around the middle indicates that there may be more fat around the organs than is healthy. A healthy WHR for women is under 0.85 and men under 0.9.

Men: chest and waist measurements. For men, the chest is an area worth measuring. More overweight men have 'moobs' now, however you can dramatically reduce chest measurements with regular exercise. Especially when you embark on a weight lifting programme – incorporating press ups (push ups) can dramatically change the shape of a man's chest. It is a good measurement to take, and combined with the waist measurement (taken around the naval); it can be an indicator of overall health. It is healthier to have a chest larger than waist. What often happens is an excess of fat on both waist and chest. The belly may in fact be larger than chest, especially if too much beer is regularly consumed. As you get fit, you lose body fat, and both chest and waist size shrinks. After developing a good fitness level, you may feel confident to start lifting weights – hey presto! Chest measurement increases as pectoral muscles develop strength. So the chest measurement may come down, and then go up again.

Finally, blood pressure, what *does* it measure?

Your heart pumps blood to all parts of your body through arteries. When your heart beats and a surge of blood is pushed through your arteries, the pressure against your artery walls is at its highest. This is called the systolic reading (the higher number of the two). When your heart is at rest between beats, this is the lowest pressure, or diastolic pressure.

Your blood pressure reading always shows both your systolic and diastolic blood pressure, the systolic (larger number) over the diastolic (lower number).

Your blood pressure varies throughout the day depending on your level of activity and / or emotions (i.e. nervousness temporarily increases blood pressure). However, overall you have an average resting blood pressure, which is why you are seated when you have your blood pressure measured.

An overall higher blood pressure reading means that your heart has to do more work to get the same amount of blood to your extremities. Not only this, but your arteries have a harder time as there is more internal pressure on them. This can lead to the walls of your blood vessels thickening to deal with the increased pressure. A thickened blood vessel wall means less blood can get through. High blood pressure can lead to stroke, heart attack, heart failure or kidney failure.

Blood Pressure Measurement

	Systolic	Diastolic
Low	< 90	< 60
Normal	120 – 140	60 – 90
Above Average	140 – 159	90 – 94
High	160 +	95 +

If you have high blood pressure, or are keen to keep yours at a healthy level, there are a number of lifestyle aspects to consider:

Salt – Reduce the amount of sodium that you consume. Studies have shown that an increased consumption of salt leads to higher blood pressure in many individuals. Salt causes our body to retain more water. In turn this extra water in our blood vessels can increase blood pressure (as there is more liquid being pumped through). Excess salt can also damage kidneys, which remove sodium from the body.

Exercise – getting regular exercise can help lower your blood pressure. Regular pulse raising activity exercises your heart, the most important muscle in your body. Many athletes have a low resting heart rate and low blood pressure as they regularly train their body to deliver oxygen more efficiently around their bodies, thereby moving more efficiently and breathing more effectively. Measured aerobic exercise is a very effective way to lower your blood pressure.

Alcohol – excessive alcohol consumption (14+ units alcohol) can cause an increase in blood pressure. Increased alcohol consumption also leads to increased weight, and so the individual has more physical bulk to carry about.

Give up smoking – a fairly obvious one.

Cholesterol levels – Cholesterol can build up in blood vessels and cause a restriction to the amount of blood that can be pumped through. If you have high cholesterol levels, a high blood pressure can prove fatal.

Stress levels – Do you have a stressful job? Or are you always worrying about something? Stress levels may lead to an increased blood pressure.

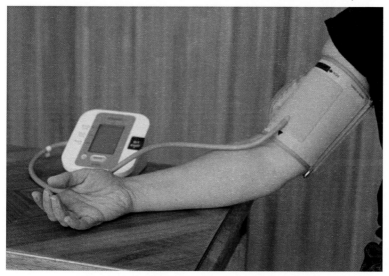

BP is a super important, but often overlooked, measurement. Many people have high blood pressure without realising it. Stressful lifestyle and too much caffeine can push your blood pressure up worryingly high. Your BP will probably be higher at the end of a working day, than at the beginning. The ideal time of day to take your own BP is in the morning, when you have woken up. This should give you the lowest reading. In fact, if you take your own BP whilst still laying in bed (prone) it will be even lower. If you're concerned about your BP, it may be worth investing in your own Blood Pressure Monitor. They're only about £20 from any pharmacy or online; industry-standard is the Omron brand. Watch a YouTube clip of how to use the cuff (or read enclosed directions), and write down your readings with the date, time of day and any incidental observations (i.e. if stressed at work).

You can experiment with taking your BP before and after coffee, or alcohol, or exercise. Alcohol and stimulants push up your BP, whereas exercise lowers it. You may also find your BP is higher when you're feeling under the weather. A higher blood pressure means there is more pressure on the arterial walls – it basically makes your life more difficult. Lowering your BP can help avoid all sorts of health implications, and can also avoid your GP putting you on blood pressure medication.

If you want a lower BP reading when you go to your GP, walk or cycle there. It should be lower after exercise. 'White Coat Syndrome' can be also common, even in the studio I find sometimes a higher reading at the first session (when the client may be initially apprehensive or nervous) than when someone is more comfortable with the environment. This is another good reason for getting your own BPM, as you can tell your Doctor what your readings at home are. They will probably be lower than the readings at the GP surgery. And that's an interesting thing that you learn, that your blood pressure is not constant throughout the day, it fluctuates, sometimes a great deal. It depends on what situation you're dealing with. Stuck in a traffic jam? Your BP may be high! The old saying 'it made my blood boil' may not be taken literally, but figuratively it's an interesting concept.

Something you may not have thought about with fitness coaching...

By looking at fitness as a puzzle, it means that when you meet someone for the first time, you pick up information on the puzzle. So much of human interaction is unspoken; it's how the body moves: our body language. How we carry ourselves posture-wise can say a lot about what is going on inside that person. I like to watch how people move as it shows a lot about their strength and particular body weaknesses.

A fitness studio can seem like an intimidating place if you're not familiar with it. I try to make the Griffen Fitness studio as comfortable as is practical, so newcomers feel welcome. House plants, a lack of heavy equipment or machines, and a few cushions, some background music – it's more like a lounge room than a studio. And that's how I like to look at fitness. You don't need to go to a place to exercise. It is incidental, something that you can do at home. I used to cycle to client's homes, getting them fit from their living room with minimal equipment. Things have come full circle and more people realise that they do not need to go to a dedicated shared space (i.e. a gym) to get fit. Gyms are great if you use the pool, lift heavy weights, or enjoy classes. If you're just looking to learn how to keep fit by yourself, you can use your immediate environment. In fact, you don't need any equipment at all if you understand a bit about how you're put together. Being naturally curious will help you on your journey of figuring out how to workout autonomously.

You also don't need fancy clothing. Fast wicking material is better than cotton (as it draws sweat away from the body, and also dries quicker). Wool is a fab textile to wear when exercising in winter. Wear clothes you're comfortable in. Some people find going out and buying new fitness kit motivates them. It's good to feel happy with what you're wearing (i.e. don't wear your oldest t-shirt if you're self-conscious about running, buy a fast-wicking running top and feel happy about looking good). You want to make it easy to get fit, and you'll be spending more time exercising, so perhaps thinking about what you're going to wear will make the experience more positive. There's a great selection of 'activewear', from M & S and the High Street, to the boutiques of Sweaty Betty & Lululemon. I often wear clothes from outdoor shops, like Trespass (excellent fleeces) or Tiso (Edinburgh). For ladies, a well-fitting sports bra is also a must for your bust. Get fitted, as you need it tighter than your usual bra. Shock Absorber is a reliable bra, and for the larger ladies, Bravissimo (Edinburgh) comes recommended. It will make everything more comfortable.

When it comes to shoes, you can wear pretty much any trainers. If you have any knee or ankle issues, you may wish to look at getting a new pair. The type of trainer you get depends on what you want to do. If you'd like to run, some cushioned running shoes make running on tarmac easier on the legs. The amount of cushioning you get also depends on your choice of activity; running shoes have more cushioning than walking or hiking shoes. Some people never plan on running, so for them buying running shoes is unnecessary.

There is a growing trend for 'fashion' trainers – Converse, Adidas, Sketchers, Vans are all fashion brands. The trainers are usually fine to exercise in. Converse 'Chuck Norris' basketball shoes are almost like minimal trainers, in that they have minimal cushioning. They're excellent for doing balancing exercises (and skateboarding!), but may not have enough cushioning if you're planning to run.

So work out what you're going to wear, first step of the plan.

It is always good to have a plan, something to guide you step by step through a process.

To get fit, you need to challenge your body in different ways. Getting your heart rate up, with aerobic (or cardiovascular) exercise helps to burn body fat, it boosts your metabolism and mood, burns calories and also gives your heart a good workout. Strength training will also help boost your metabolism, as it builds muscles. Strength training is basically putting your muscles under some sort of resistance, whether its weights, rubber resistance bands or even using your own body weight as resistance, for example press ups. Muscles are metabolically active tissue (i.e. they need calories to exist), whereas fat is stored calories. So you burn body fat with cardio exercise, strengthen and tone your muscles with strength exercise. Muscles need looking after when they've been worked, so stretching is the third type of exercise you need to do regularly. Flexibility exercises will stretch out the muscles, which helps them recover from exercise; it feels good and helps your posture too. Yoga is a good example of stretching. The more the energetic yoga is (e.g. power yoga), the more likely it is to incorporate cardio and strength. You're looking to get a balance of all three types of exercise that will help you become trim, taut and bendy! I like to start with the easiest to do... walking.

2. Introducing Aerobic Exercise

Cardiovascular, or aerobic exercise, is where you get your heart rate elevated for a period of time. Aerobic exercise varies in intensity, from low to high, with different effects. We'll start with low level intensity, for a number of reasons:

If you get your HR (heart rate) up to a level that you're slightly puffed, but not absolutely exhausted, and hold it there for half an hour or more, it burns body fat effectively and boosts mood and metabolism. HIIT (High Intensity Interval Training) does have its merits, however it's safest to start with a lower level and improve aerobic fitness before 'beasting' it. Also, it is absolutely acceptable to have a fitness programme that uses only lower level heart rate training. In other words, you don't need to do HIIT unless you really want to!

Getting your Heart Rate (HR) up so you feel puffed for 30 minutes (or more) will improve your fitness and endurance. Using a Heart Rate Monitor (HRM) is a very good way of ensuring that you are operating with your HR in the correct zone. Too many people start too fast and put themselves off exercising. Start easy and build up from there.

For many people fast walking will get them into the correct HR zone. If you're fitter, you may need to jog or even run. You can also go swimming, cycling, dancing, or anything that gets your HR elevated. Enthusiastic house cleaning or gardening could count as cardio, as long as you kept it up for 30 minutes or more.

Most HRM's will calculate your HR training zone for you, or you can use the table below. As you get older, the HR that you need to go at gets lower. For example, if you're 30 years old, 130bpm – 170bpm is your target HR training zone, for 40 years old it's 117bpm – 153bpm, for 50 years 111bpm – 145bpm.

I find these numbers pretty accurate to work with, as the fitter you are the lower your resting HR, so you will need to do more work to get to the zone. The zone is 65% to 85% of your MHR (Maximum heart rate = 220 – your age), dropping with age as per formula. Here's the table:

Heart Rate Training Zones

Age	65% (aerobic)	75%	85% (anaerobic)	Age	65% (aerobic)	75%	85% (anaerobic)
20	130	150	170	44	114	132	150
21	129	149	169	45	114	131	149
22	129	149	168	46	113	130	148
23	128	148	168	47	112	130	147
24	127	147	167	48	112	129	146
25	127	146	166	49	111	128	145
26	126	146	165	50	111	128	145
27	125	145	164	51	110	127	144
28	125	144	163	52	109	126	143
29	124	143	162	53	109	125	142
30	124	143	162	54	108	125	141
31	123	142	161	55	107	124	140
32	122	141	160	56	107	123	139
33	122	140	159	57	106	122	139
34	121	140	158	58	105	122	138
35	120	139	157	59	105	121	137
36	120	138	156	60	104	120	136
37	119	137	156	61	103	119	135
38	118	137	155	62	103	119	134
39	118	136	154	63	102	118	133
40	117	135	153	64	101	117	133
41	116	134	152	65	101	116	132
42	116	134	151				
43	115	133	150		65+ aim for 100 - 130bpm, or so you feel slightly puffed		

Once you have worked out the Heart Rate Training zone for your age, set up your HRM. I used to use an entry level Polar HRM that cost around £30 – they were excellent devices as you could set them to beep if you were outwith the HR training zone. Sadly Polar stopped manufacturing them, so an affordable alternative is the Beurer branded model, PM25. You can buy it online if you search 'Beurer HRM PM25'.

It is hugely helpful to use a device that will tell you your heart rate as you go along and let you know (via a beep or vibration) whether you are going too slow or too fast. You need to keep your HR elevated, so you are not beeping, continually for half an hour or more. The most reliable HRM's have a chest strap that pick up the electrical impulse of your heart and transmits it to a wristwatch.

There are many Activity Monitors on the market that calculate your HR by using an infrared sensor at the back of the watch, measuring the pulse in your wrist. Activity Monitors are not as accurate for heart rate training, as your heart rate varies, so it's preferable to measure your HR at the chest / heart (rather than wrist). Activity Monitors also do not have a beep, and from experience I know the beep is very handy in helping maintain the correct pace.

If you can't find a HRM with a beep, you can use a FitBit or Garmin activity monitor, just keep an eye on your HR and be aware that there may be a lag in your heart rate reading.

If you're not ready to invest in fitness technology, simply wear a watch with a second hand (or use the stopwatch function on a smartphone). You can manually check your pulse by placing two fingers (your index and middle fingers) flat against the side of your throat, just beside your oesophagus, or windpipe. You should feel a pulse, if not, then move your fingers, flat around your neck until you feel it. It may take a few attempts, and note that the higher your heart rate, the easier the pulse will be to find.

When you've perfected the method, you can briefly stop moving, and count your pulse beats for 10 seconds timed on a stopwatch or watch. Multiply the number by six, and you have calculated your beats per minute. 20 beats in 10 seconds is 120bpm, which is the lower aerobic heart rate for those who are in their mid thirties. You can refer to the chart on page 25 to find your lower limit in relation to your age.

It's logical that we don't want to go too slow, but why the upper limit? The upper HR (85%) is your 'lactate acid threshold' calculated for your age. In other words, it's where aerobic exercise becomes more difficult, or higher intensity. Your lactate acid threshold is simply where your body goes from using a mainly aerobic system in the body (i.e. using oxygen as fuel with stored body fat) to anaerobic (in extremis, where you use more stored muscle glycogen as fuel). This is not a bad thing, it's just your body using more of a different fuel (aerobic uses more body fat, anaerobic uses more stored muscle glycogen). If you are pre-diabetic, getting your HR up to a high intensity, in a safe and controlled way (i.e. on an exercise bike), can help deplete your muscle glycogen – effectively using more stored blood sugar and therefore dropping your blood sugar level.

If you are deconditioned (unfit), your HR will leap up higher and quicker when you exercise, just because you're not used to it. The more cardio exercise you do, the better trained your cardiac muscle (your heart) becomes. The stronger your heart, the more blood that is pumped each heart beat and the lower your heart rate will be.

Cardiovascular exercise is basically strength training for your heart muscle. As an added bonus it burns body fat as a fuel (keep it slow and steady) and has been proven to boost mood. LSD training (Long Slow Distance, or keeping your heart rate in the aerobic training zone) for half an hour or more has been proven to release serotonin and endorphins, like dopamine in the brain. If you think about how good you feel when you've climbed up a big hill, this gives you a good example.

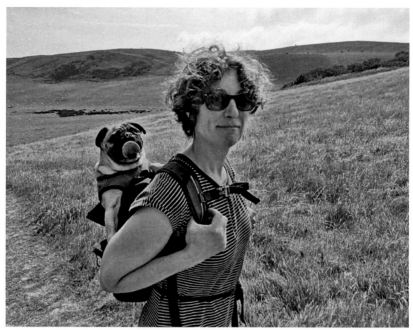

If you have a small dog you may need to be inventive... Here the author is carrying Coco the fitness pug in a backpack designed for carrying dogs – adding weight to a backpack will make walking more of a workout!

The idea is to get your HR elevated for half an hour three times per week. You can do longer and more often, but 3 x 30 minutes per week is the bare minimum. If you've not exercised much, fast walking will probably get you into the training zone. But wear a HRM, as you'll pretty soon have to start walking faster, and perhaps even jogging down the hill if your HR drops down. If you have knee or lower leg issues, fast walking may not be an option. In this case, perhaps swimming or cycling (or exercise bike, that you can hire easily) may be a better option for you.

It's important to plan your cardio sessions in your diary so they actually get done. It should be enjoyable and at a pace where you can chat (but not too easily), so plan some routes that take in local greenspaces. Look online, searching 'walks / runs near me' for ideas. Initially leave a rest day in between each session, as your leg muscles will need time to recover. You might start with walking and then discover after a few sessions, that your HR is dropping down as you walk downhill. When this happens, you'll need to do a gentle jog to push it up again. This is how we get into jogging. You'll want to do a stretch at the end, read on...

3. And Strrrrrrretch

After cardio is an ideal time to stretch. This is an invaluable skill to learn, as regular stretching eases muscle soreness and can help avoid injury.

Flexibility, or stretching, is one of the three types of exercise you need to do regularly (cardio and strength are the other two). Stretching needn't take long, no longer than ten minutes, and doing it at least three times per week will help improve your posture and range of movement. Stretching helps you recover from a workout by lengthening the muscle fibres. It also feels nice!

Stretching doesn't really burn many calories, nor does it boost your metabolism, but it does mean you recover from workouts more quickly, so theoretically you can fit more workouts into your week.

Muscles need to be pliable to be in good condition, and stretching actually lengthens muscle fibres on a microscopic scale. If you have a stretching routine, you will notice any niggles and therefore be able to address them, so they're less likely to result in injury. Stretching at the end of your workout is a good time to assess how your workout has gone, how you feel, and if there's any areas that need attention. It's also a great way of getting your heart rate down if you've been out and about.

Here's how to stretch:

1. Perform stretching exercises after exercising as your muscles are more pliable when warm. You should always stretch at the end of your workout, and you can also do brief stretches at the start, after a warm-up. The 'pre stretch' after warm-up is to prepare your range of motion, so is mainly dynamic stretching (stretching with moving, i.e. shoulder circles).

The stretches illustrated in the following pages are static stretches (i.e. holding a position) and are done for 30 seconds or more, as part of a cool down. These should be 'deep' stretches, and initial tightness will gradually diminish as you hold the stretch – holding the stretch for longer will increase your flexibility and lengthen your muscles. The larger the muscle group, the longer they will take to stretch.

2. Perform these stretching exercises after workouts, and preferably at least three times per week. You can do stretching exercises every day if you wish. It's easiest to do the floor exercises all together, as they are listed here.

3. Ease slowly in and out of the stretch. Do not bounce! Start the stretch easy and breathe deeply as you develop the stretch.

4. If you feel any pain whatsoever... stop, or lessen the stretch. Listen to your body. Tightness can indicate that extra stretching is required.

Lying Leg Stretch

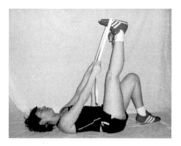

This is one of my favourite stretches that I do at the end of a busy working day. I keep a yoga belt on my coffee table so I remember to stretch if I'm watching TV. If you don't have a yoga belt, you can use a long scarf, a towel or even a no-longer-required business tie. My grandma Jean used to tell me that elevating the leg was very good to let the blood drain out and relieve sore or tired legs (good for varicose veins).

Stretches the large group of muscles at the back of your legs (calves and hamstrings) and is excellent for relaxation.

1. Lie on floor on your back, legs bent and with feet pointing forward.

2. Bring one knee in towards your chest, loop a band/ towel around the ball of the foot, then straighten the leg away from you. Push your heel towards the ceiling.

3. Pull slightly on the band/towel to increase the stretch (whilst keeping arms and hands relaxed).

4. Keep your neck relaxed, gaze to the ceiling and extended leg straight. If leg is bent, decrease the stretch slightly to straighten it. Think about straightening the knee and pushing your heel to the ceiling.

5. Hold for time required whilst maintaining steady breathing. You should be able to increase the stretch after about 20 seconds – very rewarding! You can hold for as long as you want, up to 3 minutes each leg.

6. Repeat for other leg.

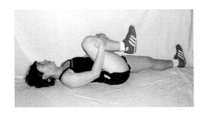

Glute Stretch

Doing this stretch lying on your back gives you the added bonus of a back stretch, which is also nice on the shoulders, especially if you've been stooped over a laptop all day.

Stretches your bottom muscles (gluteus maximus) and promotes a stretch in your back.

1. Lie on your back with your body in a straight line.

2. Breathe out as you place hands onto upper shin and bring one knee into your chest.

3. Increase the stretch by pulling knee in further whilst extending the other leg straight out in front of you. Keep your neck relaxed, your head on the floor and feet flexed.

4. Hold for time required whilst maintaining steady breathing. You can do ankle circles with the top ankle in both directions to ease any tension.

5. Repeat for other leg.

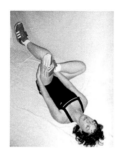

Outer Thigh and Hip Stretch

This is an essential stretch if you sit for a living (i.e. desk based work). Sitting a lot can cause tight hips, that can lead to niggles when running. You can also do this from a seated position.

Stretches the muscles in your outer thigh and into the side of your hip.

1. Lie on your back with knees bent and both feet on the floor.

2. Raise one ankle to the opposite knee, as pictured.

3. The knee with ankle on is pulled toward you, whilst the other knee pushes out. If you can't reach around your thigh, try using a band or belt around the thigh and pulling in.

4. Keep head and neck relaxed and feel the stretch in the outer hip area.

5. Repeat for other leg.

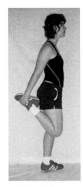

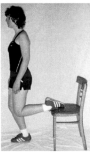

if you cannot reach to hold your foot, try the stretch with a chair

Quadriceps Stretch

Another essential stretch for desk jockeys (office based work), you can ideally do this stretch daily. It can be done lying down, and is also a handy pre-stretch for runners.

Stretches the group of muscles at the front of your thighs, quadriceps. This exercise also develops a good sense of balance. You can do this lying down, on one side.

1. Stand with your legs hip-width apart.

2. Bend one leg backwards. Reach behind with the same hand and hold the top of your foot, or even grab your ankle.

3. You can hold onto something for balance, but ensure that both of your knees are together. Pull foot towards middle of butt, and poke the hip bone forward thus lengthening from the top of the leg.

4. Ensure knees are together, bent knee pointing down.

5. Hold for time required whilst maintaining steady breathing.

6. Repeat for other leg.

Calf Stretch

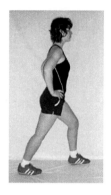

A basic stretch that can be done pushing against a wall, tree or bench. Step back further to increase the stretch. Calves tend to get tight if you're increasing walking / running pace or distance, and they're also prone to cramping (hydrate well if you experience cramps).

Stretches your calf muscles at the back of your lower leg.

1. Stand with feet hip-width apart and parallel. Take a small step forward.

2. Lean into the front foot and push into the back heel. The back leg should be straight with heel on the ground.

4. To increase the stretch, push your back heel to the floor and push hip of back foot forwards to lengthen the leg.

5. Hold for time required whilst maintaining steady breathing.

6. Repeat for other leg.

Upper Body Stretches

You can stretch your upper body whilst sat at a desk, and regular stretching can help improve your posture too.

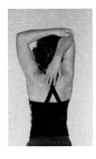

Triceps Stretch

Stretches the muscles in your triceps (back of upper arm) a.k.a. bingo wings.

1. Bring one arm above your head, and then bend at the elbow. Pat yourself on the back. Elbow is pointing towards the ceiling, and lower arm is relaxed against the back of the neck.

2. Use the other hand to gently pull on elbow. Keep neck relaxed and stance comfortable.

3. Hold for time required, whilst maintaining steady breathing.

4. Repeat for other arm.

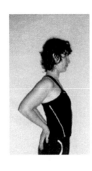

Chest Stretch

To open the chest, excellent if you've been typing on a computer all day.

1.   Stand with your arms at your sides and your feet hip-width apart.

2.   Extend both arms behind your back and place the palms of your hands on the small of your back, with fingers pointing downwards. Keep your tummy in and your eyes to the front.

3. Gently pull the shoulder blades and elbows together. Take a deep breath and enjoy.

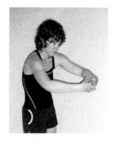

Upper Back Stretch

This stretch targets a group of muscles particularly vulnerable to tension and stress - the neck, back, and shoulders.

1. Stand with your feet hip-width apart, your knees straight but not locked, and your fingers interlaced, palms facing towards you.

2. Extend your hands in front of you, forming a large circle (like you are hugging a tree).

3. You may feel a stretch in your neck and upper back and along your shoulders. You can look towards the floor to lengthen and stretch your neck.

So get outdoors and get your HR up (cardio), then when you get home, find a space in your lounge room and do the above stretches. Get in the habit of this, and then all that's left to do is strength...

4. Strength Training

Strength workouts have traditionally been associated with going to the gym, but you can easily do these exercises from home or outdoors.

Get the Cardio and Stretching going regularly for a week or so before...

I like to introduce the strength exercises after a week of cardio and stretching. It's easiest to start with fast walking / slow jogging and stretching, and to feel the benefit of both of those types of exercise before introducing the dozen or so strength exercises to be learned. I believe in 'layering' information. That is starting small, and adding layers of complexity to an exercise programme as you go. Rome wasn't built in a day, as they say, so it takes awhile to learn and get into a regular exercise programme.

As exercising takes up a certain amount of time, it's best to fit in the 'easy' stuff first. After all, it's pretty easy to start the cardio when you have a HRM telling you what pace to go at. The trick is to get in the habit of getting your heart rate up every other day, or at least three times per week. Schedule it as an appointment in your diary, and on the day, write it on your 'to do' list (if you have one), so you can get the satisfaction of crossing it off. I have a theory that if it's not on my list of things to do, it won't get done. It's all about getting in the habit of the cardio and stretching, before we add in the strength.

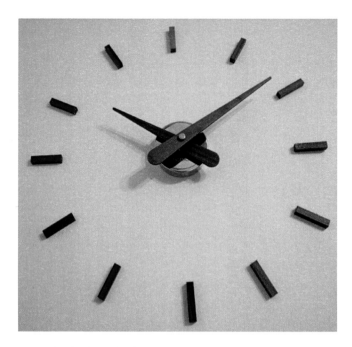

Get in the habit of scheduling your exercise in your diary,

to make sure it happens.

By the end of chapter five, you'll have the basic programme. That is, getting your heart rate up every other day (cardio), stretching your muscles every other day (flexibility) and giving your muscles a challenge under resistance (strength). By doing these three types of exercises, every other day (or more) your body will adapt to a more active lifestyle. This is what getting fit is all about, it's just a matter of the body adapting.

If you think about it, your great-grandparents would have had a more active everyday life than you, just getting things done. House cleaning was more manual, we used to carry groceries from shops (or grow more of our own food), more people walked rather than driving. Our modern lives are extremely sedentary, so an exercise programme is designed to ensure you get enough movement in your everyday life to stay in tip top shape. We're not designed to sit on our derriere all day. Sitting is very bad for your cardiovascular health and overall body (tight hips, shoulders, lazy abdominals etc).

And now, Strength

With strength training we start with exercises that use no equipment, just your own body. Bodyweight exercises are fab, as you don't need any equipment to do them, so there's never an excuse not to exercise! Gyms are becoming outdated, nowadays it's about using your body, rather than machines, to get a good workout. You may find you learn more about your own anatomy when you learn these exercises. I have to say that studying anatomy piqued my interest, the body is a fascinating thing.

On the following pages you will find diagrams of the major muscle groups. You don't need to memorise them, but you might find it handy to refer to the illustrations of where the muscles are, when you try the exercises.

MAJOR MUSCLE GROUPS FRONT

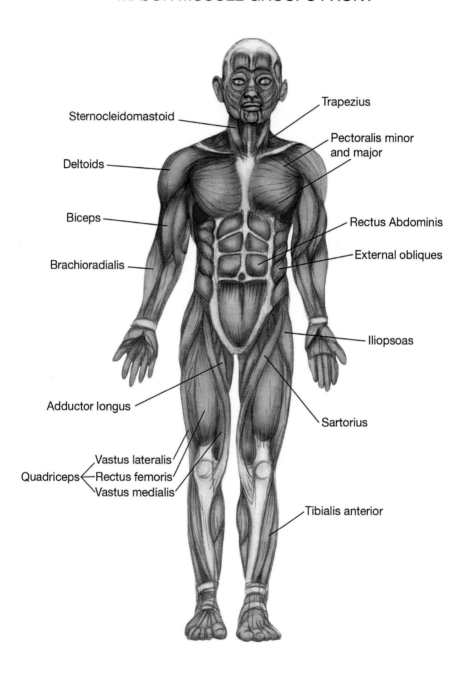

Sternocleidomastoid

Deltoids

Biceps

Brachioradialis

Trapezius

Pectoralis minor and major

Rectus Abdominis

External obliques

Iliopsoas

Adductor longus

Sartorius

Vastus lateralis

Quadriceps — Rectus femoris

Vastus medialis

Tibialis anterior

MAJOR MUSCLE GROUPS REAR

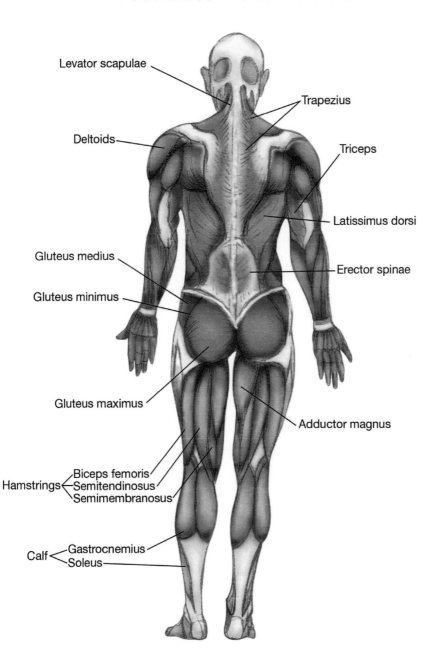

Levator scapulae

Trapezius

Deltoids

Triceps

Latissimus dorsi

Gluteus medius

Erector spinae

Gluteus minimus

Gluteus maximus

Adductor magnus

Biceps femoris
Hamstrings—Semitendinosus
Semimembranosus

Calf—Gastrocnemius
Soleus

Once you've got the hang of the basic bodyweight exercises, we can add variations. Then to get more variety we can add equipment, however it's not essential. We're going to start with upper body and leg exercises. In a separate section we look at abdominals. You can learn them separately, but then try them together. Combined, these 11 exercises form the basis of your strength programme. Aim to do this three times weekly, with rest days in between. Once you're familiar with the strength programme, together the exercises will take around half an hour. If you're doing it in under 30 minutes, try slowing the reps down.

So let's start with the basics.

Firstly, you need to warm up. Warming up need only take about five minutes, and it's designed to get your heart rate up, get oxygen pumping to the muscles, and get them ready for action. You can use your cardio exercise as a warm-up, and structure your workout: cardio, strength, and then stretching.

It might take longer to warm up on a cold day or in the morning, it depends on the individual. In the studio we'd do a basic circuit of a minute of various actions. My personal favourites are:

Jogging / marching on the spot.

Star jumps, or low impact variation.

Leg curl, kicking one butt cheek then the other with alternate heel, arms swinging forward and back.

Clapping under the knee. Stand with feet hip-width apart and arms out to the side, as you lift one knee up high, clap your hands underneath. Swap legs, so you are swinging your straight arms out to the side (parallel to the ground), then clapping under the alternate knee that is lifted up.

Or even some enthusiastic house cleaning!

Stepping: if you don't have a step at home but live in a flat, you can always run up and down the stairs for a bit.

Rebounder: if you have a wee trampoline they're fun to use in a warm-up, but not essential.

Skipping rope: one minute and build up from there. Best done outdoors, or in a large ground floor space.

A good warm up will use both the upper and lower body to warm you up quicker. You'll know you're warmed up as your heart rate goes up, you will feel warmer (you may want to take layers off) and should feel ready for action. The fitter you are, the more energetic a warm up is required. If you're deconditioned (not so fit), just marching on the spot with swinging arms may be enough to warm you up.

Sets and Reps:

Usually strength exercises are broken up into x number of sets, of y number of reps (repetitions), for example 3 sets of 10 reps = 30 reps. 30 reps is a good place to start. We're not doing loads of reps, so you can focus on your form for every single repetition. As you develop strength, you can add more reps. You can also advance the exercises by choosing a more challenging exercise variation (for example, if you are strong already, you may wish to start with full press-ups. For those not exercising, starting with the box press up is a good idea).

It is good to think about the muscle group you're targeting as you exercise, as this has been proven to make the exercise more effective. If you think about your quadriceps (front of thigh) as you squat, it has been scientifically proven that more blood will flow to the area and more muscle fibres will be engaged. To find out more about visualising muscles engaging, look online for 'motor imagery'.

Try these initial five exercises in the order listed. The workout starts with three variations of press ups. Read through them then choose the press-up option suitable for your current fitness level. Then follow with triceps dips, squats, lunges and buns of steel.

You can do abdominals straight after, or try the core exercises after a breather.

If you have any questions, or need some guidance, I offer webcam sessions to teach the strength exercises.

Press Up / Push Up (standard) Variation 1

This classic bodyweight strength exercise is excellent for your chest. It's a pushing movement, as if you were pushing yourself up off the floor. Most people start with the box position (knees under hips), and as you get stronger you can take more of your body weight forward into the intermediate position (with flat back).

If you have had a knee replacement, or struggle to get down on the floor, try press ups standing up against a wall (next exercise).

To work chest and back of the upper arm.

1. Start on all fours, knees hip-width apart and hands slightly wider than shoulder-width, tummy tucked in. Your eyes should be looking at the spot between your hands to keep your neck long.

2. Breathe in, bend at the elbows and slowly lower your nose to floor. The intermediate position has a flat back and your chest coming down to the floor.

3. Breathe out, straighten arms and push yourself back to starting position, whilst still keeping tummy tucked in.

- do three sets of ten reps, the further you take your weight forward, the more difficult.

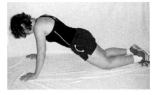

Box position

(less weight forward)

Intermediate position

(more weight forward)

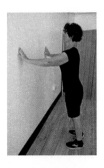

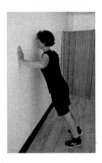

Press Up against wall (easier) Variation 2

This is an excellent variation if you are unable to kneel. The further you take your feet from the wall, the greater the angle and therefore the more difficult. Start quite close to the wall!

To work chest and back of the upper arm

1. Stand a short distance from a wall, hands on the wall, slightly wider than shoulder-width and *at chest height*, back straight and tummy tucked in.

2. Breathe in, bend at the elbows and slowly lower your chest to wall.

3. Breathe out, straighten arms and push yourself back to upright, whilst still keeping tummy tucked in.

- do three sets of ten reps, at least three times per week.

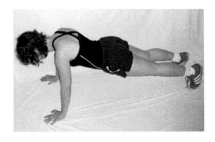

Full Press Up (advanced) Variation 3

This is the advanced version of press ups (or push ups), that people imagine themselves doing. It's actually quite tough, and you need to build up your upper body strength by doing the easier variations first. Choose this level if you have already been doing strength training or if you are confident that you can keep good form. You'll also need good core (abdominal) strength, just to hold the position.

To deeply work pectoral (chest) muscles, also arm and shoulders.

1. Start on all fours, with hands wider than shoulder-width, back straight and tummy tucked in. Raise yourself onto your toes, making sure your back is straight and not dipping down. Your hands are quite wide.

2. Breathing in, bend at the elbows and slowly lower chest to floor whilst looking down and keeping neck long. See how low you can go.

3. Breathe out, straighten arms and push self back to starting position, whilst still keeping tummy tucked in.

- do three sets of ten reps at least three times per week *superslow*

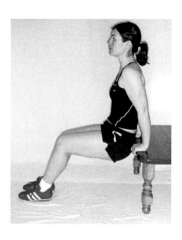

Tricep Dips

This is a tough one, but I like to teach it at the start as it is very satisfying to see the 'bingo wings' tone up. You will feel this one maybe two days after, so be sure to stretch at the end.

If you are a bit on the heavy side, this may feel impossible to start, but it will get easier with practise! It will also strengthen your wrists.

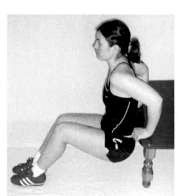

You can do this on your sofa at home. If the sofa is too low, try it on the arm of your lounge suite. If they're too high, use a sturdy coffee table, blanket box, or any heavy piece of furniture that is high enough for you to take your weight off of, but so that your thighs are about parallel to the ground when you start. You knees should be around 90 degrees and feet hip-width.

To strengthen and trim triceps (back of arm).

1. Sit on the bench, hands either side of you.
2. Shift your weight off the bench, so your straight arms are supporting you, elbows are pointing directly backwards, fingers pointing forward towards you.
4. Breathe in and bend the elbows, lowering your rear down. Point your elbows back behind you. Your rear end should stay close to the bench, so bend elbows loads!
5. On the exhalation, straighten your arms, thereby lifting you back up to the start position. You can progress this exercise by positioning your feet further away from you.

- do three sets of ten reps at least three times per week. If you're struggling, you can start with sets of five reps and build up from there.

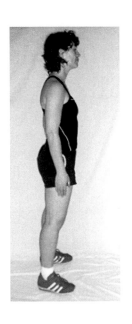

Squats

The classic leg strength exercise, this is an example of functional fitness as it is effectively a 'sit to stand'. Being able to stand up unassisted from a seated position enables ease of movement. There are many variations of this exercise that we will look at, once you've mastered the standard squat.

Works the front (quadriceps) of the legs as well as the bottom muscles (gluteals)

1. Start with feet hip-width apart, tummy in and back straight.

2. Tuck your abs in, push your bottom out and down into a squat (as if you were sitting on a small chair). Your weight goes into your heels, and move arms out in front of you to help balance.

3. Lower your hips down. The end position is with thighs around parallel to the ground (or as close as you can). You will find your squats get deeper with practise.

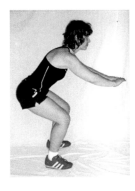

4. Breathing out, straighten legs and return to starting position. Knees are relaxed at the top and do not 'lock'. Tuck your bottom under to complete the movement. By squeezing your butt and back of thighs as you stand up, you lengthen the legs without locking the knees.

- do three sets of ten reps at least three times per week. You can also break them into two sets of fifteen (my personal preference).

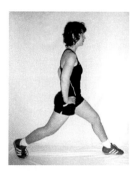

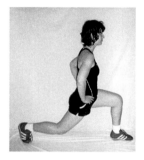

You can use a chair back for support.

Lunges

Another classic leg strength exercise, this works your hill walking muscles. You can also work this muscle group by walking up stairs two at a time. This is also a good way to strengthen knees and challenge your balance.

Works front of the thigh (quadriceps) as well as a bottom muscles (gluteals)

1. Start with feet hip-width apart and tummy tucked in.

2. Take a big step forward. Your step forwards needs to be big enough so that the back heel is up. Ensure feet remain hip-width and back heel is elevated.

3. Breathing in, bend the back knee toward the floor in a downward motion (not forward).

4. You should always have an angle of ninety degrees or more in the front leg.

5. Slowly exhale and straighten the back leg, returning to the starting position.

- do two sets of ten reps at least three times per week.

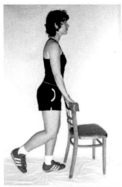

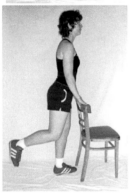

'Buns of Steel'

This is a lesser known exercise but I like to include it early on in the programme as it can be done anywhere, anytime. It's a good one to do when you're boiling the kettle for a cuppa. The important thing is to keep the top half of the body still, so you're just working the butt muscles.

We sit on our gluteus maximus all day, so it's important to give it a dedicated strength exercise. Did you know your glutes are the biggest muscle in your body? Even standing up to work can help tone the glutes. Sit less, stand more.

Works the bottom line of the rear muscles (gluteals)

1. Start with feet together and tummy tucked in. Lift one leg up, bent behind you with foot flexed.

2. The supporting leg is also slightly bent (i.e. knee not locked).

3. With a small movement, move your elevated thigh back, squeezing the rear end.

4. Keep the bend in the knee frozen, it is only your glutes doing the movement, not your knee. The thigh bone squeezes back, then returns to the midline.

If you feel any cramping in the back of the leg (this is common), bring your knee up towards your chest to stretch it out, then continue the set, remember to breathe. If you feel pain in your lower back, pull in your tummy more and focus on the leg kicking back.

- do two sets of ten reps at least three times per week. Build up to two sets of twenty reps.

Well done!

You can now try abdominals. The previous strength exercises are movement-based exercises. Core strength has a different emphasis - many abdominal exercises are static, holding still, to work deep muscles.

There's some theory to digest before moving onto tummy work. Grab some water and read on. If you choose, you can leave abs for another day and instead stretch to finish off your workout. It's up to you.

5. All About Your Abdominals

Your abs are in your torso, also known as core muscles. A strong core means better posture, a smaller waistline, less lower back pain and an overall improvement in quality of life (you can do more. I like to work abdominals separately from the rest of the body, as there's quite a collection of muscle groups in your abs, and they all perform a different function. For a comprehensive abs workout, you really need to work them for their purpose, which means having a fair selection of exercises to play with. The Pilates exercise system does exactly this – named after exercise pioneer and guru Joseph Pilates (1883 – 1967 it exercises all three groups together to improve posture and get rid of belly bulge.

Rectus Abdominus – superficial

Superficial muscle groups are on the outside and help your body move. In the case of your rectus abdominus, or six pack, they flex the spine (bringing the rib cage closer to the pelvis) and are used in the abdominal crunching / sit up movement. As they are a superficial muscle group, if you have low body fat, you can see a toned six-pack.

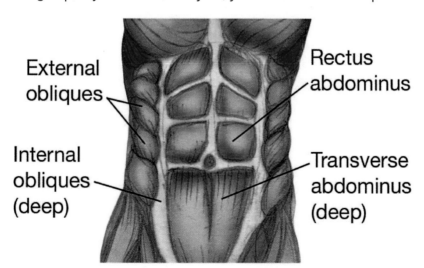

External obliques

Rectus abdominus

Internal obliques (deep)

Transverse abdominus (deep)

Transverse Abdominus – stabilising

This is the deepest abdominal muscle group – deep muscle groups such as these are postural and help keep your body in place as you move. In essence your deep abs work by holding you still. The plank (in the following workout) is a good example. In Pilates the transverse abdominus is known as 'the girdle of strength' as it acts as a natural belt, keeping your insides in and is essential for trunk stability. This is the muscle group that is important to exercise and strengthen, as it is a deep muscle group often not exercised in movement based programmes. Moving works your superficial muscles, holding still works your deep, postural muscles.

Pilates exercises focus very much on using traverse abdominus to build 'core strength'. Some people find that developing core strength supports their back and alleviates lower back pain. One of the causes of lowerback pain can be weak abdominals, meaning your lower back does more work, and then complains about it by hurting.

Internal and External Obliques

Your internal obliques are deep muscles on the side that stabilise your spine as you twist and rotate. External obliques are on the outside, as the name would suggest. They're your 'love handles' and assist in side bend movements.

How to locate your transverse abdominus

In a kneeling position, press your fingers below your belly button and cough. One of the muscles contracting, the transverse abdominus, stabilises your spine because it's the deepest of the abdominal muscles. It wraps, sort of like a corset, from the bottom of your rib cage in the front to the ribs in your back and holds the visceral organs in place.

Learning how to engage your transverse abdominus (getting into 'neutral spine')

It's good to 'engage your abdominals' at the start of every tummy exercise as it helps get your abdominals ready for action. The action of engaging your abs involves positioning your spine in its natural curve, neutral spine, and then sucking your belly button in tight. Here's how to do it from a lying position:

1. Lie on your back with your knees bent and feet on the floor, hip-width apart.

2. Press your spine to the floor so that it's completely flat against the ground.

3. Now curve your spine up away from the floor so there is space under your lower back.

4. Do this several times, making the movement smaller and smaller until you have reached the midpoint. It should feel comfortable.

5. Hold this position. Place both thumbs on your belly button and make a triangle with your fingers pointing down to your pubic bone. This triangle should be flat, and if someone balanced a glass of water in the middle of this triangle, you shouldn't spill a drop!

6. Stabilise this position by imagining zipping yourself into a tight pair of jeans. The muscle contraction is both in and up, as if 'zipping up' from the pelvic floor under the waistband.

7. It will take time and practise to learn to stabilise these muscles, but once you've got the hang of it, your waistline will thank you.

On the following pages you will find the introductory abdominal exercises. The lower abdominal exercise to start is very much a focussing exercise, you're concentrating on locating where these deep core muscles are, and holding them in. The more you do it, the more of the deep core muscles you will be able to engage and the stronger your core will become.

It's worth spending a bit of time getting to know these exercises and what they do. Some people find it tricky to get these muscles working, and that's not unusual. We spend much of our days slumped at computers, so we need to teach our postural muscles what to do. Have patience and persevere and you will get the hang of it.

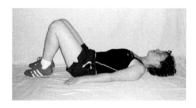

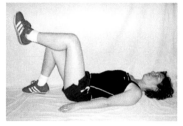

Lower Abdominal Exercise – raising leg

A Pilates exercise to isolate and engage deep abdominal muscles. As you're working deep muscles, the aim of this is to keep your tummy as still as possible. Imagine you have a very full glass of water balanced on your tummy. You don't want to spill it, so keep your tummy tucked in for the full two minutes. Use a stopwatch.

1. Get into neutral spine - Lie on your back with knees ninety degrees, feet hip-width flat on the floor, abdominals pulling in and arms relaxed by your side. Focus on a spot on the ceiling directly above you and breathe naturally into your chest.

2. Slowly raise one leg, until the raised shin is parallel to the floor.

3. Breathing out, gently lower leg back to the floor. Whilst lowering down concentrate on keeping your abs flat and as still as possible. Keep your hip bones still, do not allow them to rock from side to side.

4. Repeat for other leg and keep pace slow.

- do *two minutes*. With practice you will find that you can pull in even more of your tummy muscles the longer you go.

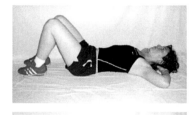

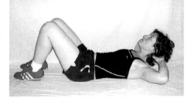

Abdominal Lift

A neck-friendly version of the crunch, this works the rectus abdominus. Your 'six pack' muscle group is a movement muscle group, flexing your spine (the lift). You should feel this in your upper abdominals, not your neck.

1. Lying on your back with legs ninety degrees and tummy held in, in neutral spine and with your hands behind your head. Focus on a spot on the ceiling directly above you and *keep your elbows back.*

2. Contract your stomach (upper abdominal muscles) and breathe out to lift your torso upward. Beware of pulling on your neck and keep your eyes to the spot above you so your neck remains long. Slowly lift to as high as is comfortable.

3. Breathe in on the way down and repeat.

- do twenty reps at least three times per week.

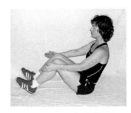

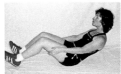

Abdominal roll down

Works the deep abdominal muscles, the 'muffin top' area just above the waistband. These muscles support your lower back, so if you feel any discomfort in your lower back as you roll down, lessen the movement and pull your tummy in more.

1. Sit with legs bent, feet flexed and arms stretched out to the front (as per diagram).

2. Sit up as straight as you can.

3. Tuck your abs up and under to start the slow roll down.

4. Lower down a short distance, and then back up again. Keep your shoulders and arms relaxed so your abs does all the work.

5. Keep breathing and focus on pulling in the abdominals whilst you roll slowly up and down. It doesn't matter how far down you go, as long as you feel it in your lower abs.

- do ten reps slowly up and down.

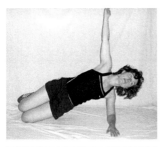

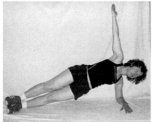

Side Plank

Works the obliques (love handles)

1. Lie on your side, lining up your knees with your hips and shoulders along a straight line. Your elbow should be directly under your shoulder.

2. Pull up to your knees so the side of your torso is lifted off the ground (as per top photo)

3. The more advanced level is the bottom photo, lifting up onto feet. Stack the feet on top of each other, and it's easier with shoes on (but definitely possible barefoot).

- Try fifteen seconds on each side and build it up as you like.

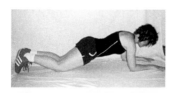

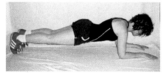

The Plank

Works the transverse abdominus muscles, this is a classic exercise that can be done anywhere anytime. If you're unsure, start with the first level to knees. Be sure to pull in your tummy and breathe!

You don't need to hold it for ages, the most important thing is to have good form. The longest you really need to plank for is a minute (build up to it).

1. Lying on your front, straighten up, prop yourself up on your elbows, keeping your tummy tucked in and your neck long (eyes look between hands).

2. Raise yourself up so that you're now propped up to your knees (or feet, more advanced lower photo). Ensure that your lower back is lengthened, bum down and tummy pulled in. Push through your heels and squeeze your butt.

- do thirty seconds.

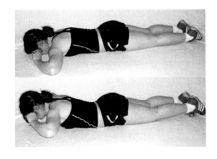

Back Extension

Works the erector spinae, lower back muscles – just above the waist band. If you work your front, it's good to work your back too.

1. Lie on your front with arms bent and fingers to temples. Tuck your tummy in and make sure you're lying straight.

2. Looking at the floor and breathing out, lift your torso by contracting the lower back. Keep it smooth, slow and small to start.

3. Breathe in on the way down and repeat. You can do whatever breathing you find most comfortable... as long as you are breathing!
- do two sets of ten reps.

These six exercises, with the five upper and lower body strength exercises, form the basis of your new strength programme. Do them three times a week. In the long run, you can do them more often if you wish. But you will see the benefits if you do them every other day for the next month.

It's good (at least to start with) to have a rest day in between strength workouts. This is because it's in between workouts that your muscles get stronger. Doing resistance work puts your muscles under strain, causing microscopic tears in the muscle fibres. It's the healing of these fibres, bigger and stronger than before, that develops your strength. You need time for the muscle fibres to heal before putting them under pressure again. You might feel muscle soreness to start with, this is DOMS. Delayed Onset of Muscle Soreness sometimes occurs a couple of days after a strength workout. It's a sign that the muscles were challenged.

Triceps especially seem prone to DOMS. Have a rest day with some stretching, and then do the exercises again. Whilst some muscle pain is normal, extended or acute pain should be addressed.

The good news is, the more you do, the easier it gets. Your muscles adapt. As you get stronger, you can then advance the workout.

So from week two you have: cardio (30 minutes in the zone) three times a week, stretching after workouts and strength three times per week. You can do the cardio and strength on the same day, or separate days, as you wish.

Some people like to do strength Mondays, Wednesdays, Fridays and cardio Tuesdays, Thursdays and weekends. Work out what works best for you.

It's good to look at the three types of exercise (cardio, strength, stretching separately to start with, so you know what you're trying to achieve with each. It may feel like a lot of start with... However, now we've got the constituent parts, we can start to combine exercises and multitask (which will save time and add variety.

6. Combining Cardio and Strength in an Outdoor Circuit

So far we have looked at the three types of exercise separately. They are:

1. Cardiovascular exercise (aerobic): Exercise that gets your heart rate up, using body fat as a fuel and boosting your metabolism. Aim to get your heart rate elevated so you feel slightly puffed but not absolutely exhausted, for at least 30 minutes continuously, at least three times per week. at least three times per week. You might find that you're already going faster for longer, and with less effort. The more you do, the easier it gets as your body adapts.

2. Strength exercises (anaerobic): Putting your muscles under some form of resistance, using either your body weight (no equipment, just your body) or equipment (that we will look at in the next chapter). This makes muscle fibres denser and more numerous - overall stronger and more defined. It will also boost your metabolism, as muscles need calories to exist, even at rest.

3. Flexibility exercises (stretching): Static deep stretches are done at the end of a workout, when the body is warm and muscles more pliable. This will improve your flexibility, posture, aids cool down and relaxation and also feels good. It can also help you avoid injuries by stretching out tight bits.

To do cardio and strength well, you generally need to spend around half an hour on them each. Many of us are pushed for time, so you can combine the cardio and the strength in an outdoor circuit. All you need is some greenspace with benches and a heart rate monitor (or a method of checking that your heart rate is 'in the zone').

You can start your workout the moment you leave your front door. Do this by walking or jogging to your local park to get your heart rate in the training zone, starting slowly to warm up. You should have worked out your ideal pace by now. Aim to move at a pace that feels sustainable for a while. If you're getting too puffed, slow down a bit. We can look at higher intensity cardio a bit further down the line. For the time being, a fast walk or slow jog should suffice.

The idea is to use the trip to the park as your warm-up, getting your HR elevated and blood pumping around the body. When you get to the park, we can get straight into some strength exercises.

For this workout you're keeping your HR elevated for at least half an hour (cardio), whilst doing your upper body and leg strength exercises (strength): exercise multi-tasking. At the end of the workout, head homewards to do abdominal exercises indoors, as your HR will drop down. Most days in Scotland the weather is not great for lying down in a park, so try prone (lying) exercises indoors, as part of the cool down. All of the outdoor strength exercises are done standing up, as they will keep your heart rate up.

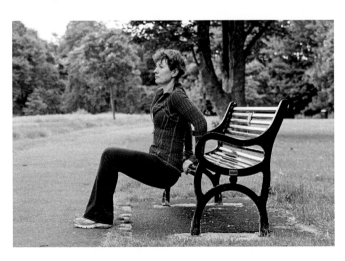

In the park, locate a suitable bench, and do triceps dips on the front, and press-ups on the back of aforementioned bench, as per previous photo. You can alternate sets between press-ups and dips, rather than do all three sets together (i.e. 10 of each alternating). You might find that your HR drops down as you do the strength exercises, so the idea is to use different benches between sets to keep your HR up. Do a set of 10 press ups on the back of a bench, then 10 triceps dips on the front, and then quickly move onto another bench for the second and third sets.

You will also find that if you can use a bench up a hill (i.e. you're fast walking / jogging up the hill before doing the strength) that it will push your HR up for the start of the strength (where it will drop down again). You may also find that triceps dips pushes your HR right up to start with, but as you adapt to the strength exercises, it's less of an effort, so less of a 'shock' to the body, and less likely to push your HR up. Be sure NOT to sit on the bench between sets, as your HR will drop down. The idea is to keep your HR up, so you need to keep moving, while keeping good form.

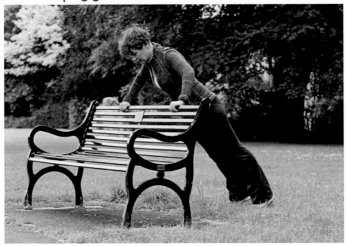

A word about standing press-ups on the back of a bench. Use a wide hand grip (as pictured), and bring your chest to the back of the bench. You can bend slightly at the waist to make it easier. The more upright you are, the less resistance (or weight) going through your chest. So to make it more challenging, have your feet further back and your body straight. By doing them upright it keeps the HR up. If you get down onto hands and knees on the ground, you will notice your HR drop down. The idea of this circuit is to keep your HR up and do the strength exercises, so no resting in between sets. This is where a HRM is very useful. I like to start with the upper body, as most people find it the most difficult. We use our legs to walk around, so they have some inherent strength. Most people don't lift or carry stuff and have poor upper body strength. So whilst triceps dips might feel like the most difficult exercise, they're also the exercise where many people see the most improvement (and toned upper arms, bye bye bingo wings). Press ups and triceps dips are the proverbial bread and butter of upper body strength – the two main exercises without equipment that work the top of the body. You will find as you progress, triceps dips get easier, to the point where they don't push your HR up. In that case, you may want to start a cardio / strength workout leg exercises. Your legs have bigger muscles in them than your arms, so exercising your legs usually gets your HR up more than exercising your upper body.

To continue, fast walk or jog to a scenic part of your favourite park, I like to exercise out of the way of major thoroughfares, usually with my back to a hedge or wall. This is because when you do squats (that's next in the strength programme), you want to stick your bottom right out behind you. If you're at all self-conscious face away from a blank surface (i.e. have your back to a fence or wall), so you can really sit down into the squat without worry.

As an aside, it's worth pointing out the practicalities of exercising in a public area. Pick your favourite benches and spots in the park, and that becomes your new gym. Some areas of the park are busier. If you stick to quiet spots out of people's way, it makes for a more relaxing workout. If you're exercising on the path, be sure to leave space for people to walk past and remember you may have friendly dogs coming up to say hello as you workout – it's their park too!

Once you've got your HR up again, stop and do 15 squats, then 10 lunges on each leg. We're going to look at a couple of variations for the second set (buns of steel to come). If your HR has dropped down, then fast walk / jog to another spot. The second set is a set of 15 plies, and 10 striding lunges.

The exercises are illustrated on the following pages.

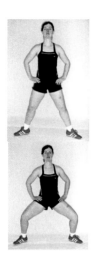

Plie Squats

A squat variation, out-turned feet works more lateral thigh and hip muscles, on the side. Excellent for quadriceps strength and also knee robustness.

1. Start with feet very wide apart, toes pointed out at 10 o'clock and 2 o'clock, bottom tucked under and back straight.

2. Keeping yourself upright (as if sandwiched between two pieces of glass) push your knees outwards and down whilst lowering down into a wide squat.

3. Squeeze the back of your legs back up to the starting position, adding in a squeeze of the rear near the top for added value.

4. Knees are relaxed at the top and do not 'lock'.

- do one set of fifteen reps.

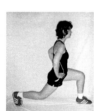

Striding Lunges

Works front of the thigh (quadriceps) as well as bottom muscles (gluteals). They have the added bonus of pushing your HR back up.

1. Start with feet hip-width apart and tummy pulled in. You can put your hands on hips.

2. Breathe in and take a big step forward. In the same movement, bend your back knee down into a lunge. The weight stays over the back foot, so it's a lunge down, not forward.

3. Breathing out, push back, straightening your leg and stepping back to the start position.

4. Repeat, alternating legs.

- Try ten reps on each leg.

The plies help work more lateral leg muscles, and the turned-out foot position engages different muscles from a standard squat. Striding lunges are more explosive and will also push your HR back up. Unlike in a gym, the outdoors can have an uneven surface, and sometimes it's even windy, which means you have to keep your balance.

So by doing a variety of exercises outdoors, you use a lot of different muscle groups, which helps with balance and proprioception (that's awareness of the position of the body).

The last exercise to be done outdoors is buns of steel, so fast walk / jog to another bench. Hold onto the back of bench for support. You'll find that standing on one leg whilst doing buns of steel keeps your HR elevated, something to do with how the heart pumps blood around the body (i.e. it's more difficult for the heart to pump blood when you are standing on one, rather than two legs, so your HR goes up). Handy for doing single-legged exercises and these exercises are also excellent for keeping your legs injury-free.

As you ramp up your fitness it's important that you remain injury-free. An injury is a major reason many people fail on an exercise programme.
Start easy, and build up as your fitness improves. There is little benefit from 'beasting' yourself, you're more likely to get injured and put yourself off. Start easy and enjoy your workouts and you'll find yourself actually wanting to exercise. It's fun designing your own circuit in your local park or back garden.

I personally find an outdoor workout is one of the best mood boosts around. You're getting your HR up, breathing clean air, releasing endorphins, viewing a far horizon (rather than a screen, or walls), increasing your Vitamin D intake, interacting with nature whilst strengthening your body. What's not to like?

And the next chapter is about the fun of introducing equipment. Even if you stopped here, you are now equipped to create your own exercise programme. All you need to do is get your heart rate up every other day, give your muscles a challenge every other day, and then stretch them out... Every other day!

Enjoy!

7. Adding Equipment

It is absolutely possible to get fit without using any equipment. Simply use your body weight for strength, cardio and stretching. However, adding simple equipment can offer you a broader variety of exercises that will work a variety of different muscle groups, in different ways. To recap:

For anyone walking or running on tarmac, a comfortable pair of shoes is essential. Cushioned running shoes can help absorb the impact of jogging on hard surfaces. If you're running off-road, cushioning is less important, but support might be useful. So buy a shoe to suit what you're doing. You don't need to spend a lot, but a new pair of shoes can feel amazing and help motivate you to exercise (we all like wearing new shoes!). If you develop sore shins when you start running, the first thing I'd do is look at your shoes. It may be a result of shin splints, which can be caused by increasing either mileage or pace too quickly, or from impact, so cushioned footwear can help. Also running off-tarmac, on grass or sand helps avoid sore shins.

You will have noted that early on I recommended investing in a HRM (Heart Rate Monitor). This is excellent to help you undertake aerobic exercise at the correct intensity level. As you get fitter, your heart rate is lower, so you'll need to exercise at a higher intensity to enter the cardio 'zone'. You can wear an activity monitor if you wish (Fitbit, Garmin etc) with a HR display. It might not be as responsive as a HRM with a chest strap (it won't be as accurate either), but some people like to record their daily activity. Personally I find the concept of a third party holding information about my heart rate over the day, a bit worrying. In July 2020, a certain activity monitor platform was hacked and users ousted for three days. In the future, activity monitors may be used by life insurance companies. Just imagine that...

For ladies, a supportive well-fitting sports bra is a bust must. You want something that really straps you in! The less bounce, the easier it is to move. If you're blessed in the chest department, you may need to look around for a decent option. I prefer non-underwire, as bra underwire can interfere with a HRM pick-up (wire crossing the chest strap confuses the device).

These are things that are definitely worth investing in. Now, to add variety to your strength exercises, we can look at the following equipment:

Dynaband, also known as a Pilates band: this flat latex band offers a natural resistance that is inexpensive, portable, versatile and robust. They are often used for physiotherapy rehabilitation exercises. Latex-free options are available for those with a latex allergy. There are different strengths of band, usually starting with green or yellow for easy (injury rehabilitation), blue is usually mid-strength and then you have the tougher bands that are red or black. I usually use a 1.32 metre long blue band. Keep your band out of direct sunlight to avoid perishing, and check it for damage before use.

The following band workout is an alternative strength workout to your bodyweight exercises; in that it's a whole body workout. It's especially good for shoulders, legs and deep abdominals. It's an excellent workout for a dreary day outside. Just grab a glass of water, put on your favourite music and clear some space in the lounge...

Dyna Band Exercises

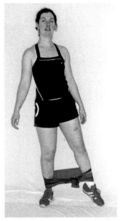

Warm up with blue band

To warm up and strengthen the inner / outer leg and knee muscles, do around ten reps of each exercise listed below. Keep tension in the band at all times. This prevents it from falling down and gives your legs a better workout.

Good music with a strong beat is helpful. Rather than counting reps, you may prefer to do the workout to your favourite music. Do a move for verse, another move for chorus etc. Improvise!

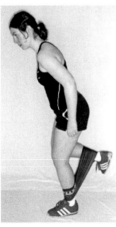

Tie the band in a loop around your ankles, with feet hip-width apart. Tie ends in a bow, so it is easy to untie.

- Side Step, stepping side-to-side keeping tension in the loop at all times. Swing your arms and find a side-step rhythm. One foot steps sideways, then the other one follows.

- Toe point, with feet hip-width apart, point big toe of one foot to the front, alternating feet.

- Heel Dig, with feet hip-width apart, tap one heel to floor at the front, alternating feet.

- Do a Leg Curl, bend the knee, bringing your heel toward your rear, like you're trying to kick your butt. Keep your feet wide.

- Double Step, like side step but with two steps to each side, keeping tension in the band.

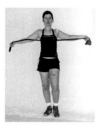 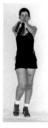

Chest Flye

Shapes and tones the chest muscles (pectorals).

1. Stand tall with the end of the band in each hand, arms straight and band flat across the back.

2. Bring the arms together at the front, arms straight.

3. Return to start position.

4. You can march on the spot to keep your legs moving.

- do three sets of ten reps, slowly.

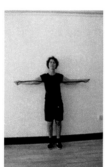

Shoulder Press

Strengthens and tones the shoulder muscles (deltoids).

1. Stand tall with the end of the band in each hand, arms straight and band flat across the back. It's the same start position as for Chest Flye.

2. Bring the arms up above your head, keeping arms straight and band securely anchored under shoulder blades (beware of 'pinging' yourself with band as you lift arms up).

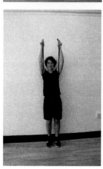

3. Return to start position, making sure arms do not drop below parallel to the ground, or the band may lose its anchor point on your back.

4. You can march on the spot to keep your legs moving.

- do three sets of ten reps, slowly. You can alternate sets of Chest Flye / Shoulder Press for variety.

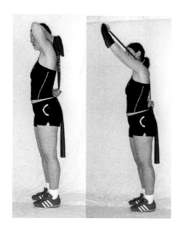

Tricep Extension

Works the back of the upper arm (triceps), the same muscles used in triceps dips. If you struggle with dips, try this option. It works both sides of the body separately – most of us have a dominant arm, and it can be quite different between left and right.

1. Hold the end of the band in one hand. Raise the arm, pointing toward the ceiling, then bend at the elbow and let hand fall to behind the neck.

2. The top arm is arm bent with elbow next to your ear, pointing to ceiling. Hold the other end of the band with your other hand in the small of your back so there is some tension.

3. Extend the top hand toward the ceiling, keeping your elbow high and near your ear in a Tricep Extension.

- do three sets of ten reps on each side, slowly.

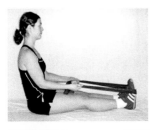

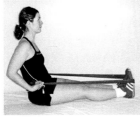

Low Row

Works the mid back (latissimus dorsi) and is excellent for posture.

1. Sit on the ground with legs together and straight out in front. Wrap the band around your feet, halfway down (around instep) and sit up straight, holding the ends in each hand.

2. Keeping the elbows tucked in tight, pull the ends of the band towards your hip bones in a Low Row.

3. Think about pinching the shoulder blades together and sitting tall.

- do three sets of ten reps, slowly.

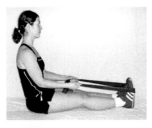

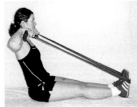

High Row

Works the upper back, between the shoulders (rhomboids and latissimus dorsi)

1. Sit on the ground with legs together and straight out in front. Wrap the band around your feet, halfway down (around instep) and sit up straight, holding the ends in each hand. It's the same start position as for Low Row.

2. Poking the elbows out to the side, pull the ends of the band towards the front of your shoulder.

3. Think about pulling the elbows out to the side and sitting tall.

- do three sets of ten reps, slowly. You can alternate sets of Low Row / High Row for variety.

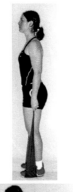

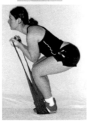

Squat with band

Works front of the thighs (quadriceps) as well as bottom muscles (glutes), and you can also get your upper arms (biceps) in on the action too. This will get your heart rate up as you use both upper and lower body.

1. Stand on the middle of the band, feet hip-width apart, holding each end of the band.

2. Engage your abs and push your bottom out down into a squat. Your weight goes into your heels.

3. At the same time, pull up on the band by bending your elbows, keeping them tucked in tight to your sides.

4. Breathing out, straighten legs and arms, returning to starting position. Knees are relaxed at the top and do not 'lock'.

- do three sets of ten reps.

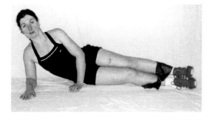

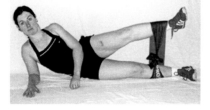

Outer Thigh Raise

Works the side of the butt (gluteus medius), outside thigh and knee. An excellent running strength option.

1. Start by lying on your side in a straight line. You can prop yourself up onto your elbow if you wish. Have the band looped around your ankles.

2. Breathing out, lift your top leg with heel flexed, stretching the band loop. Keep the foot parallel to the ground to work into the outer thigh.

3. Keep your foot flexed, breathe in and lower. Keep tension in the band.

- repeat slowly for twenty on each side.

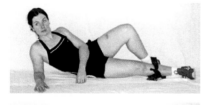

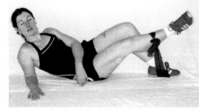

Inner Thigh Raise

Works the inner thigh (adductors) and is good for overall leg strength.

1. Start by lying on your side in a straight line. Place the foot of your top leg on the floor behind your bottom calf. The back foot stands on the loop of the band, anchoring it to the ground behind the straight leg.

2. Breathing out, lift the straight leg with heel flexed, whilst making sure your tummy is tucked in. Keep your foot parallel to the ground.

3. Breathe in and return to the ground.

- repeat slowly for twenty on each side.

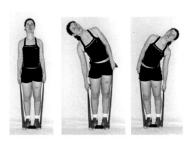

Side Bends

A brilliant toning exercise for the external obliques, 'love handles'. It's also a nice stretch for the back and can feel quite relaxing.

1. Hold the end of the band in each hand and stand in the middle, feet hip-width apart. You want a lot of tension in the band for this exercise.

2. Imagine you are sandwiched between two panes of glass, so you can't sway forward or back.

3. Staying 'sandwiched', lower one hand down one thigh squeezing into the side bits. Let your head relax with the movement.

4. Repeat for other side.

- do fifteen reps on each side at least three times per week. You can also try this with dumbbells.

Abdominal Roll Down

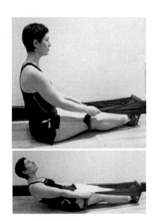

Works the deep abdominal muscles

1. Sit with legs straight, feet flexed and arms stretched out to the front holding onto each end of the band, which is around your feet.

2. Sit up as straight as you can.

3. Tuck your abs up and in to start the slow roll down

4. Roll down a short distance, then roll back up again. Keep your shoulders and arms relaxed so your abs do all the work.

5. Keep breathing and focus on tucking in the abdominals whilst you roll slowly up and down

- do ten reps slowly up and down, then four holding for four counts as low as is comfortable.

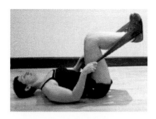

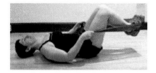

Lowering Legs (Knees bent)

Working into the deep abdominals, the trick to this is to keep your tummy squeezed in and your back in neutral position. Try not to arch your spine, and if you feel discomfort in your lower back, make the movement smaller.

1. Lie on your back, loop the band around both feet and bend your knees at ninety degrees to your body.

2. Slowly push your thighs away from your body with feet moving towards the floor. Keep your knees frozen at ninety degrees.

3. You should feel this in your lower abs, so pull in tight under your waistband. If you feel it in your lower back, lessen the movement and pull your tummy in even more.

- Try twenty repetitions.

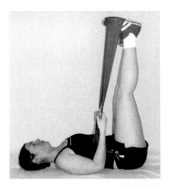

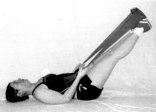

Lowering Legs (Straight), Advanced version

Similar to Lowering Legs (Bent) on page 82, but more challenging. Only try this if you have a good degree of abdominal strength - keep the movement small, and focus on pulling in the lower abdominals under your waistband.

1. Lie on the floor on your back. Holding each end of the band, loop the band around both feet and extend both feet to the ceiling, so your legs are straight at about a ninety degree angle to the floor.

2. Pull on the band, so you have a decent amount of tension in the band. Anchor your elbows to the ground.

3. Pulling in your abdominals, slowly lower your straight legs towards the ground, using the tension of the band to assist. Only go as far as comfortable, and do not go all the way down, even a little movement is good.

4. Raise your legs back to the start position.

- repeat for ten slowly, going only as far down as is comfortable.

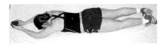

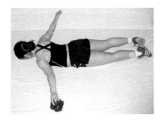

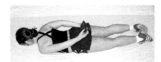

Lower Back 'Passing the Band'

Works the lower back muscles (erector spinae) – just above the hip area.

1. Lie straight on your front with your arms stretched out in front of you and legs straight. Hold the bundled-up band in your outstretched hands.

2. Breathing out and squeezing your lower back, elevate your torso off the ground.

3. Your arms move in a circular motion, parallel to the floor, as you pass the band from one hand to the other, first above the head, then behind the back. Remember to keep breathing, as you feel is right for you.

- Do ten in one direction, then ten in the other.

As the band workout is a whole body workout, feel free to have a nice stretch at the end. You can do the band workout as an alternative to your bodyweight strength programme.

When you get to know the exercises, you can combine band exercises with your bodyweight workout. Here's an example 'best of' workout:

Warm up – 5 minutes

Press ups – 3 x 10 reps

Tricep dips – 3 x 10 reps

Low row with band – 3 x 10 reps

High row with band – 3 x 10 reps

Squats / plies – 2 x 15 reps

Lunges / striding lunges – 2 x 10 reps

Outer thigh with band – 20 reps

Inner thigh with band – 20 reps

Isolating deep abdominals with leg raise – 2 minutes

Ab lift – 20 reps

Roll down with band – 10 reps

Lowering legs bent / straight with band – 10 reps each

Dorsal Raise (lower back) – 20 reps

Stretch

The band is a very easy to store piece of kit. Less easy to store, but also as useful, is what was called a Swiss ball in the 80's - now known as an exercise ball. You're looking for a ball big enough to sit on comfortably. Exercise balls generally come in three sizes: 55cm (small for shorter height), 65cm (medium for average height), 75cm (big for taller height). You can generally tell if a ball is the correct size for you by sitting on it. Your knees should be around 90 degrees, at right angles. You're not too close to the ground, nor balancing atop the ball. Also, how well-pumped up the ball is will make a difference. Lastly, the type of material the ball is made from is important. Anti-burst balls are robust, and live up to their name: not bursting. Very important. The cheap vinyl rubber balls you used to get free with a Special K™ cereal are difficult to use, and can pop. Avoid.

Just sitting on the ball will get your deep abdominals working as you need to engage your deep transverse abdominus just to stay balanced. Some people like to use an exercise ball instead of a desk chair, and it certainly does make you think of your posture. This is a more advanced workout, so feel free to just try a couple of the exercises. Balancing on the ball is a good place to begin. Start with three minutes and build up from there...

HEALTH AND SAFETY FIRST! Check the ball for damage before using. Move furniture out of the way, especially when balancing on the ball. It will make it easier for you to balance, as your peripheral vision will not have to worry about potential hazards.

If you are unsure of any of the exercises, please do feel free to contact me for assistance. I offer webcam exercise demonstration sessions worldwide, just visit www.getfitandenjoyit.com

Ball Exercises

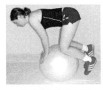

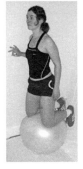

Balancing on the ball

Challenges your balance and uses all of your deep core muscles.

<u>On all fours:</u> Start positioned behind the ball, with both hands on top of the ball and knees in a square shape. Toes are still on the ground. Slowly lean forward, pushing into your hands, lifting your feet off the ground so you are balancing on top of the ball on all fours. Push your hands in to the ball to stabilise the position and hold for as long as you can! This will take practise.

<u>Kneeling on the ball:</u> The easiest way to learn this is by positioning the ball in the corner of a room and kneeling on top of it. When you have mastered this, kneel on the ball, side on to one wall. With practise you will be able to kneel on the ball in the middle of the room with no assistance from the walls... Hold for as long as you can!

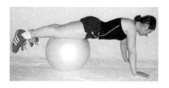

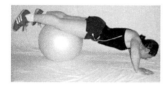

Press Ups

Works the back of the upper arms and chest

1. Kneel behind the ball, with plenty of floor space in front of you.

2. Roll yourself over the ball so you are supported by your arms with the ball under your thighs, in a press up position.

3. Breathing in, bend your arms and lower your upper body down as far as is comfortable.

4. Breathing out, straighten your arms (without locking elbows) so that you are in the starting position.

5. You can alter the difficulty by rolling yourself further from the ball (i.e. so the ball is under your lower shins or ankles). Be sure to keep your tummy in and back straight.

- try three sets of ten reps, alternating the distance of the ball.

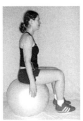
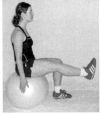

Leg Extensions

Works the front of the thigh (quadriceps) and also your deep core muscles

1. Sit on top of the ball with knees at ninety degrees and tummy muscles engaged. You can hold onto the ball if you wish, or go 'hands free' for more of a challenge.

2. Keeping one foot on the floor, extend the other leg so it is straight out in front out of you. Hold for a second, then return foot to floor.

3. Alternate leg extensions.

- do twenty reps (ten on each leg).

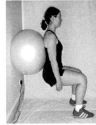

Squats

Works the front of the thigh (quadriceps)

1. Place the ball against a wall and stand with the ball between your lower back and the wall. Your feet should be hip-width apart and a fair distance in front of you, so you are leaning against the ball with diagonal legs.

2. With your tummy tucked in, bend your knees and roll the ball up your back so you sit into a squat position. Knees should be around 90 degrees and you need to lean back into the ball, with straight back.

3. Breathing out, straighten legs and return to starting position. Ensure knees are straight but do not 'lock'.

- repeat for three sets of ten repetitions.

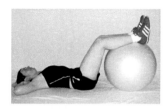

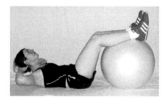

Abdominal Curl

Works the tummy (abdominal) muscles

1. Lie on your back with legs at ninety degrees, and resting on the ball. Tuck your tummy in and place your hands behind your head. Focus on a spot on the ceiling directly above you and keep your elbows back.

2. Contract your stomach (abdominal muscles) and breathe out to lift your torso upward. Slowly lift as high as is comfortable.

3. Breathe in on the way down and repeat. - do two sets of ten reps.

Hamstring Curl

Works the back of the thigh (hamstrings)

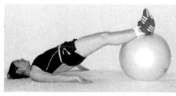

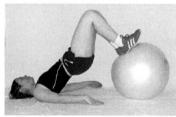

1. Lie on your back, with your heels on top of the ball and legs straight.

2. Elevate your hips so your back is off the ground and your heels are balanced on the ball.

3. Keeping your hips as high as possible, bend your knees in towards your butt. You'll feel this in your hamstrings.

4. Straighten to start position. You may feel cramping in the back of your thighs, this does happen. Relax down and bring your knees into chest and then try again.

- repeat 10 times, slowly. Build up to 2 sets.

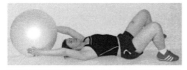

Passing the Ball between your hands and feet

Working into the deep abdominal muscles and rectus abdominus.

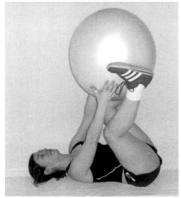

1. Lie on your back, knees slightly bent and hip-width apart. With straight arms, hold the ball on the floor, above your head.

2. Breathing in, take the ball with your hands to your middle, as your legs are also lifting up to meet in the middle.

3. Pass the ball from hands to your feet, and breathing out, carry the ball between your feet down to the ground. Keep your knees bent. At the same time your arms return back to their starting position (minus ball) above your head.

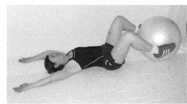

4. Breathing in and using your feet, bring the ball from the ground to your middle. At the same time, your hands are moving from above your head to your middle, where the ball is then passed.

5. Breathing out, return the ball to the starting position above your head whilst your bent legs also return to their starting position.

- do ten reps; a rep is a full cycle down and up.

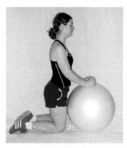

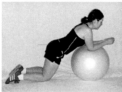

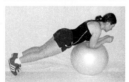

The Plank

Works deep into the abdominal stabilising muscles

1. Kneel behind the ball, back straight and fists resting on top of the ball. Lean into the ball and roll it along your forearms, so you are leaning at an angle on the ball with your stomach clear of the ball. Pull your abs in and keep your back straight. This is the half plank position.

2. When you have stabilised in this position, lift your knees so you are balancing on your toes with elbows digging into the ball. Concentrate on breathing and keeping your tummy tucked in. This is the full plank position. If you feel your lower back getting nippy, either lower your knees, or pull your abs in more.

3. To progress this exercise, when in the plank position move your elbows forward. You will feel an increase in the load on your abs.

- Try 30 seconds.

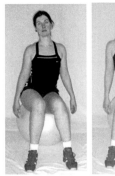
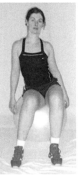

Seated Ball Swing

Works the external obliques.

1. Sit on the ball with your knees bent at ninety degrees and feet flat on the floor.

2. Moving your rear from side to side on top of the ball, squeeze into each side, thinking about bringing the side of the hip closer to the rib cage (i.e. squeezing into the love handles!).

3. Keep your shoulders still, so only your bottom half is moving.

4. After you have tried this do some circles each way.

- do twenty reps (ten on each side).

Ball Bridge

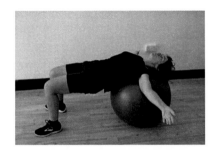

Works into the deep abdominals and tests your balance.

1. Sit on the top of the ball, with plenty of floor space in front of you.

2. Slowly lean back and shuffle your feet forward, rolling the ball up your spine so the ball is positioned under your shoulders. Position your arms straight out either side, pull your tummy in so your back is strong and lifted up.

3. You are now forming a bridge.

4. To add to the challenge try shuffling your feet to one side, rolling the ball from your spine to your shoulder.

5. Moving in a crab-like fashion, shuffle from side to side, rolling the ball from one shoulder to the other.

- Try ten reps each way.

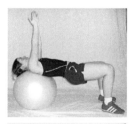

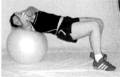

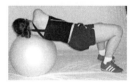

James Bond

Challenging your obliques and your balance

1. Starting in the Ball Bridge position (see page 93), bring your hands together directly above you. Your palms are clasped and arms straight.

2. Ensuring that your back is strong and your hips high, twist your joined hands to one side, rolling your shoulders over the ball. Your lower body should still be pretty much facing upwards, however your upper body has twisted 90 degrees to one side.

3. Now slowly twist in the opposite direction, ensuring that your tummy remains tucked in and your back strong. You should now be looking at the opposite side of the room.

- Repeat for ten each side, slowly and with control.

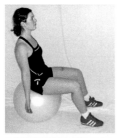

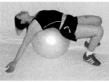

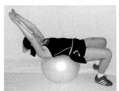

Around the World

Working into the rectus abdominus (six pack), front thigh and deep abdominal muscles.

1. Sit on the ball with your legs bent and feet flat on floor, arms relaxed by your sides.

2. Breathing in, sweep your arms out and around as you let yourself roll backwards onto the ball. Moving the ball forward with your legs will help facilitate this movement.

3. When you are all the way outstretched on top of the ball, breathe out as you sweep your hands together from above your head to a seated position, the start point.

4. Moving the ball back to the starting position with your legs will enable this movement to be nice and smooth.

- do ten reps.

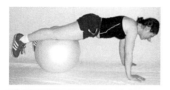

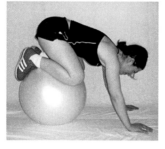

Rolling the Ball (advanced)

Working into your deep abdominals

1. Position yourself in the far press up starting position, with the ball under your shins.

2. Put your body weight into your arms, bend your knees and pull the ball forward with your shins. You will now be in a tucked up position.

3. Straighten your legs and roll the ball back to the starting position, ensuring your back remains strong (by pulling in your tummy)

- Repeat for ten repetitions in and out. Build up to two sets.

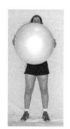

Standing Twist with ball

Works the internal obliques

1. Standing straight with feet hip-width apart, hold the ball in your hands at chest level, with arms straight in front of you.

2. Twist torso with ball to one side. Your upper body will twist and your hips should remain as still as possible. Your eyes follow the ball so head turns with the movement.

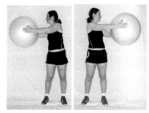

3. Only twist as far as is comfortable and be aware of controlling the movement.

- do twenty reps (ten each side).

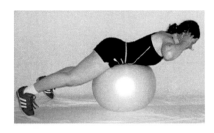

Lower Back exercises

Exercises the lower back muscles, erector spinae

Variation 1 – Back Raise

1. Face down on the ball, lie with your hips on top of the ball and your feet wide to keep your balance. Fingers to the temples and back relaxed over the ball.

2. Breathing out, raise your upper body upwards so you are now in a straight line balanced on the ball.

3. Breathe in and return to starting position.

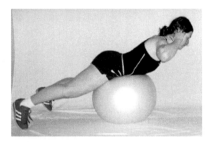

- do ten reps.

Variation 2 – Leg Raise

1. Roll yourself onto the ball, so you are face down in a near press up position. Your hips should be on top of the ball, with your arms supporting you and legs straight out behind you.

2. Breathing out, lift your legs skyward whilst keeping your arms strong (i.e. the top half doesn't move).

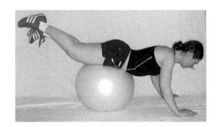

3. Breathing in, return your legs to the starting position.

- do ten reps.

Another alternative piece of kit are dumbbells. Whilst they're very popular in a gym environment, not everyone has the space to keep a full weights kit. If you do like weights, you can just use a small selection, and vary the number of reps you do for each exercise. Instead of dumbbells, you can even use a tote bag with tin cans. A bit bulky, but still a reasonable way to do strength. For chest weights a bench is essential. Most people do not have a gym bench at home, but anything that is bench shape (a sturdy piano stool, large pouffe or bench seating) will suffice. Alternatively, you can use an exercise ball as a bench (from bridge position in exercise ball workout, page 93). It is advisable to have a fitness professional show you the best form for each exercise to avoid injury and ensure correct form and speed. Start light, with 2kg or 3kg weights to perfect your form, and gradually increase your weights. You will find the bigger muscles groups (back and chest) can lift heavier than smaller groups (i.e. shoulder and arm).

You can also use filled up 500mL water bottles, obviously they are quite a lot lighter (0.5kg each) but it's a good place to start learning the movements or if you want to start easy.

Dumbbell Exercises

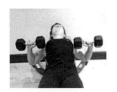

Chest Press

Similar to a press up, to strengthen chest (pectorals) and also triceps.

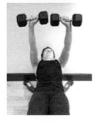

1. Lie on a bench with legs bent and tummy tucked in, hold a weight in each hand, with elbows at a right angle and at chest level.

2. Breathing out, slowly straighten arms, pushing upwards so both weights meet above the chest – the movement is in a triangle shape. Do not lock elbows.

3. Breathe in and return arms to the starting position.

- do three sets of ten reps.

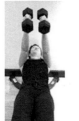

Chest Flyes

To tone chest (pectorals).

1. Lie on a bench with legs bent and tummy tucked in, hold a weight in each hand with arms extended in front of you and weights together. Do not lock elbows.

2. Breathing in, slowly bring arms in a wide arc so that arms are at 90 degrees to torso and level with chest height.

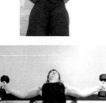

3. Breathing out, slowly return arms to the starting position.

- do three sets of ten reps. Concentrate on eliminating wobble from the movement.

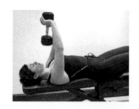

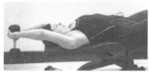

Dumbbell Pullover

An isolation exercise for the middle and upper back, latissimus dorsi.

1. Lie on a bench with your head near the end. Hold a single dumbbell in both hands with arms straight, hands overlapped and supporting the end of the weight.

2. Breathe in as you lower the weight 90 degrees to behind your head (i.e. so it is level with the bench). You will feel a stretch in your upper back.

3. Breathe out as you return the dumbbell to the start position, directly over your chest.

- do three sets of ten reps.

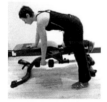

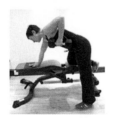

Single Arm Dumbbell Row

Tones the middle back, latissimus dorsi.

1. Rest one shin on the edge of the couch / bench and position yourself so your supporting leg is straight and out to one side. Supporting arm is straight, back flat and in the other hand is a dumbbell.

2. In a motion similar to sawing a piece of wood, breathe out, lifting the dumbbell up to your outer ribs whilst keeping the elbow in tight.

3. Breathe in as you return the dumbbell to the start position.

- do three sets of ten reps.

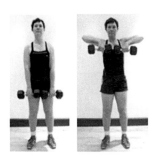

Upright Row with Dumbbells

Strengthens the trapezius (top of the back)

1. Stand with feet hip-width apart, tummy in and back straight, holding a dumbbell in each hand in front of your thighs.

2. Lift weights straight up, elbows high whilst breathing out. It's as if you're following invisible train tracks up your thighs and torso to your chest.

3. Breathe in and return to starting position. Do not sway!

- do three sets of ten reps.

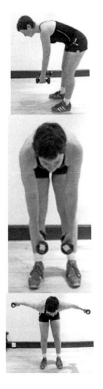

Rear Deltoid Raise

Works the back of the shoulder (posterior deltoids), an area that is often weak from slouching at a laptop. Be careful with this exercise, and do not allow dumbbells to swing.

1. Stand with feet hip-width apart, dumbbell in each hand in front of your thighs. Engage your abdominals and lean over to nearly a 90-degree angle, with back straight (check your posture in a mirror).

2. Breathe out as you lift your arms out to each side as if you are trying to take flight. The top position is with arms extended out to each side, parallel to the ground with palms facing down.

3. Think about pulling your shoulder blades together to create the lift.

4. Breathe in to return to the start position.

- do three sets of ten reps.

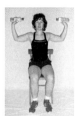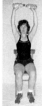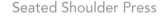

Seated Shoulder Press

Adds shape and strength to your shoulders (deltoids).

1. Sit on a seat with tummy tucked in to straighten and protect the back.

2. With a weight in each hand, arms are at ninety degrees to shoulders, palms facing to the front.

3. Keeping your back straight and breathing out, push the weights upwards to meet above your head. You may wish to use a mirror.

4. Breathing in, return to starting position. Do the whole triangle movement in a slow and steady fashion.

- do three sets of ten reps.

Lateral Raise

Shapes the side of shoulders (lateral deltoids) and arms.

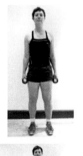

1. Stand with feet hip-width apart, tummy in and back straight.

2. Holding the weights in each hand, lift them straight out to the sides whilst breathing out.

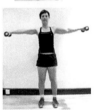

3. Breathe in and return to starting position. Do not sway!

- do three sets of ten reps.

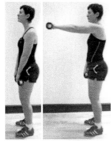

Front Raise

Works the front of the shoulders (anterior deltoids) and the tops of the arms.

1. Stand with feet hip-width apart, tummy in and back straight.

2. Holding a dumbbell in each hand, and lift one at a time out to the front whilst breathing out.

3. Breathe in and return to starting position. Do not sway.

- do three sets of ten reps.

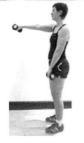

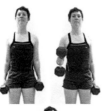

Supination Curls

Works the front of the arms (biceps)

1. Stand with feet hip-width apart, tummy in and back straight. Hold a weight in each hand with your palms facing inwards, and keep your elbows tucked into your sides.

2. With your palm still facing inwards raise one weight. About one third the way up, rotate your forearm so it is facing upwards.

3. On the way back down, do the rotation so the palm is back to facing inward.

4. Repeat for the other arm.

5. The aim of the game is to keep your elbows in tight so you work the front of the top half of your arm.

- do three set of ten reps.

In conclusion, there are oodles of strength exercises you can try, with lots of different kit. There are always new fads on the market, but when you know the basic strength movements, you will find that you don't need fads (although they can be fun for five minutes).

The type of equipment I like is affordable, portable, versatile and easy-to-store. Sometimes people are surprised by the lack of machines in the Griffen Fitness studio. Your body, my friend, is the machine! The highlights of each workout:

Bodyweight (no equipment): balance and coordination, basic moves.

Pilates band: hips and legs, abdominals, back (rowing).

Exercise ball: balance and deep abdominals, also back muscles.

Dumbbells: chest, back, shoulders and arms.

If you wish to get heavier with bulging muscles, then you may choose to lift heavier weights - a gym is handy for this. To bulk up, the general formula is to focus on strength over cardio and flexibility. Doing regular weights sessions, increasing the weight and decreasing the number of reps will make your muscles hypertrophy (grow). Use a coach, or someone who can spot your form, and please don't forget your core.

Explore all the different movements you can try. The more varied strength exercises you practise the stronger overall you will become. Don't just do your favourite exercises, as they will already be stronger muscle groups. Resistance work is meant to be a challenge, so find your least favourite exercise (often triceps dips) and OWN IT! Do it so often it gets easy. You will notice a difference.

Even a set of ten reps whilst waiting for the kettle to boil is worthwhile. Make three cups of tea in a day and you've got your squats covered. You can fit in strength exercises into your daily routine, you can do some whilst watching the television. Just go for it.

And enjoy strength, it is so good for you. You're really doing your body a favour. Remember that not every workout has to be a tough one, sometimes it's good just to go through the basics. Enjoy it, and you will find yourself looking forward to your workouts. But do it, and do it regularly – consistency is key for your muscles to develop.

8. Moving Forward

Congratulations on reaching the final chapter, I hope you have enjoyed getting into exercising... This is by no means the final chapter in your fitness journey, but just the start. In the final session (usually of a block of five) with a PT client I would do their measurements again.

You might find that some of your measurements change, whilst others take time. For instance, it is quite common for someone to lose a lot of weight quite quickly and then plateau. It's about finding a level that you're happy with. If you enjoy your fitness programme, it will become part of your life. You might cycle to pick up the groceries, walk to work, or even meet up with friends outdoors for some exercise together (hill walks with family or friends is fun). If you're feeling disheartened, consider how long it took to put the weight on – it may take a wee while to come off! Stick with it and you'll see results. Little and often is the effective way.

If you keep a balance of challenging your body at least every other day, you'll be fit and healthy. You should remember by now: get your heart rate up every other day, put your muscles under a challenge every other day and stretch them out every other day. You can do more if you like, but remember to keep a balance. We naturally prefer things we are good at, but they don't necessarily challenge our fitness. Every now and again, try something completely new – a roller blading lesson, white water rafting, disco dancing, parkour, a new hill or event. Put yourself out of your comfort zone and work towards it.

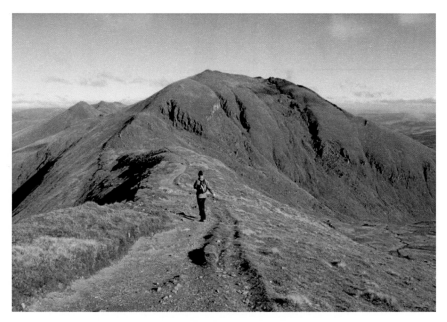

Set yourself a challenge to work towards.

In our final PT session, we would try a 'best of' workout, combining bodyweight strength with exercises with equipment (often with the Pilates band, as it is such a good, cheap and portable piece of kit), as per page number 84.

Getting started is the first step in your journey, now you have momentum it will be easier to roll with it. Rope in a friend, family member or even your dog. Remember that they may have a different level of fitness, so sometimes it's good just to work at your own pace. Homeostasis is your body maintaining its current state, it 'prefers' to stay the same. That means you do need to make changes to see changes – and also that you need to plan over a matter of months as well as weeks. You may have a dodgy week where you don't exercise as much as you'd planned to. Make a mental note of what caused this interruption and how you plan on dealing with it next time. You may choose to have certain weeks off (for example a holiday, or family visit), but always plan when you're going to get back into it.

Schedule your workouts into your diary to make sure they happen. Write your workout on your list of things to do, so you can get the satisfaction of crossing it off. Don't wait until you have a 'spare moment', or you'll never exercise at all. Make it as important as a work meeting, get it done and enjoy the results, as well as the chance to switch off your brain for a bit!

You have now put together a comprehensive exercise programme that is safe and effective. Feel free to email me if you have any questions, and I also offer webcam workouts, if you'd like to try the strength exercises with individual attention and guidance from a highly qualified and experienced Personal Trainer.

Get fit and enjoy it!

PS – Check out the 'Healthy Living Yearbook', my first book, with loads of recipes, healthy eating ideas and exercising with the seasons.

Order your copy from www.healthylivingyearbook.com, only £9.99 with free UK delivery.

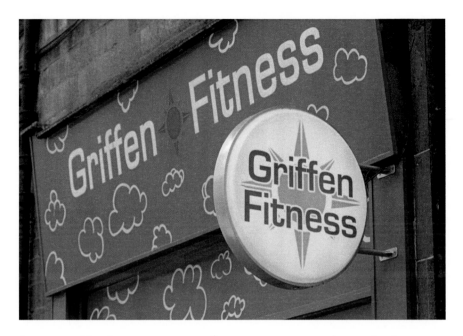

If you need further instruction, ideas or motivation, please do drop me a line, always happy to help:

www.getfitandenjoyit.com

Twitter: @tracygriffen

Facebook: /griffenfitness

Instagram: /griffenfitness

9. Recommended Reading – some of Tracy's favourite fitness books

1. 'Pregnancy and Fitness: all you need to know to exercise safely and effectively throughout pregnancy' by Cherry Baker
Excellent and easy to follow advice for Mums-to-be.

2. 'How the Body Knows its Mind' by Sian Beilock
When you move your body it affects your brain – here's how.

3. 'The Body: A Guide for Occupants' by Bill Bryson
An entertaining exploration of the human body. A long read, with lots of fascinating anatomical information.

4. 'The places that scare you: A guide to fearlessness in difficult times' by Pema Chödrön
A Buddhist text that helps with personal resilience.

5. 'Flow: The psychology of optimal experience' by Mihaly Csikszentmihalyi
The Classic text on understanding how to embrace your 'flow' state, including exercising

6. 'Healthy Living Yearbook' by Tracy Griffen
Tracy's first book published in 2011, containing 75 easy healthy recipes and seasonal exercise ideas.

7. 'A Philosophy of Walking' by Frédéric Gros
How walking and thinking are related, with beautiful illustrations.

8. 'Born to Run' by Christopher McDougall
An adventure story about the greatest barefoot distance runners on the planet.

9. 'What I Talk about when I Talk about Running' by Haruki Murakami
Prolific Japanese novelist uses running as part of his creative process.

10. 'The Obree Way: A training manual for cyclists' by Graeme Obree
For cycling geeks, this is a rare manual of unconventional advice.

11. 'Bounce: The myth of talent and the power of practice' by Matthew Syed
How to get very good at something.

12. 'Positively primal: finding health and happiness in a hectic world' by Emma Woolf
Living more naturally, close to nature.

10. About the Author

Personal Trainer Tracy Griffen established Griffen Fitness in 2005, cycling to all of her clients in Edinburgh by bike, getting them fit with minimal equipment. Griffen Fitness is now located in a private studio in Leith, focusing on fitness without using a gym. Tracy specialises in effective exercise that can be done anywhere anytime, and believes in tailoring workouts to the individual. She has a passion for the great outdoors, whether cycling, running, park circuits, or walking her studio assistant, Coco the fitness pug. The author of the Healthy Living Yearbook (2011), containing 75 easy seasonal recipes, Tracy is also a keen cook and allotment gardener.

You can book in with Tracy for a webcam workout (via Skype, WhatsApp, Facebook Messenger or Google Meet) if you'd like her to show you personally how to 'get fit and enjoy it'.

Twitter: @tracygriffen
Facebook: /griffenfitness

Sign up for her free monthly fitness newsletter, or to book in visit www.getfitandenjoyit.com

You can also email tracy@griffenfitness.com

11. Acknowledgements

Who would have thought it would take a nearly decade to write my second book? I couldn't have produced this without the help of husband, best friend and business partner Andy Wright. He took most of the photos in this book, including all of the workout photos (and he even appears on the front cover). Artist extraordinaire Rona Innes hand-illustrated the anatomical diagrams, check out her website www.ronainnes.co.uk. Thanks also to Gaby Soutar of The Scotsman for enthusing about Griffen Fitness outdoor sessions late-lockdown, leading to the quote on the cover.

Huge thanks to my proofing posse: Claire Wilson, Sharine Wilson, Sharon Wilson, Monty Roy and Alice Thomson. You made the book better. Big thanks to you, the reader. 'Get fit and enjoy it' is the approach I've used for years, and seen great success with my personal clients, so I hope you enjoy it too!